Matters of Life and Death
Key writings

Dr S MURRAY
Mackenzie Medical Centre
20 West Richmond Street
Edinburgh EH8 9DX
Tel: 0131 650 8101

Matters of Life and Death
Key writings

IONA HEATH

with a contribution from
John Berger

Radcliffe Publishing
Oxford • New York

Radcliffe Publishing Ltd
18 Marcham Road
Abingdon
Oxon OX14 1AA
United Kingdom

www.radcliffe-oxford.com
Electronic catalogue and worldwide online ordering facility.

The Mystery of General Practice was first published in 1995 by The Nuffield Provincial Hospitals Trust.

Iona Heath has asserted her right under the Copyright, Designs and Patents Act, 1998, to be identified as Author of this Work.

British Library Cataloguing in Publication Data

A catalogue record for this book is available from the British Library.

ISBN-13: 978 1 84619 096 4

Typeset by Pindar New Zealand (Egan Reid), Auckland, New Zealand
Printed and bound by TJI Digital, Padstow, Cornwall, UK

Contents

Preface

I am indebted to many people but above all to those many patients who, over the last 30 years, have taught me about different ways of living and dying and, as a result, almost everything I know about what it is to be a general practitioner.

The greatest single debt is to John Berger in both the example and inspiration of his writing and the generosity and encouragement of his letters. Much of this book arose out of the ideas and thinking that we have exchanged over several years. Very gently, he has encouraged me to search more deeply and has unfailingly provided the cues to help me think things through.

Many colleagues and friends have also helped – either through conversation or their own writing or by commenting on earlier drafts of the whole or parts of this text. Here I must mention Björn Nilsson, Per Fugelli, both Charlotte Holsts, Carl Edvard Rudebeck, Anna Donald, John Nessa, Regin Hjertholm and James Willis but there are many others.

In June 2003, I had the enormous good fortune to be invited to participate in a five-day seminar organised by Edvin Schei and the Filosofisk Poliklinikk of the University of Bergen. The seminar was held at the magnificent Rosendal estate in Norway and it was here that I was first able to try out my ideas with wise colleagues. I was immensely encouraged and helped by their response.

Finally, I thank my family – Daisy, Eric and most of all David – for their patience, their tolerance of the time it has all taken and their consistent belief that I have something to say.

Iona Heath
September 2007

About the Authors

Iona Heath has been working as an inner city general practitioner at the Caversham Group Practice in Kentish Town in the London Borough of Camden since 1975.

In 1989, she stood in the national ballot for the Council of the Royal College of General Practitioners to protest about the threat to suspend GP training in the North East Thames Region. She has been a member of College Council since then and chaired the Health Inequalities Standing Group from 1997 to 2003 and the Committee on Medical Ethics from 1998 to 2004. She is the current chairman of the College's International Committee and the Ethics Committee of the *British Medical Journal*. From 1997 to 1999, she was a member of the Royal Commission on Long Term Care for the Elderly and she was a member of the Human Genetics Commission from 2004 to 2007.

John Berger is a storyteller, essayist, novelist, screenwriter, dramatist and critic. He is one of the most internationally influential writers of the last 50 years, who has explored the relationships between the individual and society, culture and politics and experience and expression in a series of novels, essays, plays, films, photographic collaborations and performances, unmatched in their diversity, ambition and reach. In 1967, together with the photographer Jean Mohr, he published *A Fortunate Man: the story of a country doctor* which is widely regarded as quite simply the most extraordinary book ever written about general practice.

A Story

John Berger

A Story

F was 95 and, although when he walked he was as bent as a half-closed jack-knife, he still cooked his own meals, read the newspaper and followed what is happening in the Middle East. Since the death of his wife, no woman had lived in the farmhouse. His sons, who did, had enlarged the herd of milking cows from three (when they were at school) to well over 100 today. As F grew older his sons, who believed in work, accepted him as he was, and did not try to change him. He was a man who thought and prayed and did not work a lot. By temperament an anarchist. Both deferential and obstinate. Recently the sons rebuilt the entire house, but they left his room, next to the kitchen, untouched so that he could still take exactly the same steps, pursuing his routine of cutting up vegetables for his soup, praying, lighting his pipe and trying to answer his own questions.

The Tuesday before last F died. In the evening just before the milking began the sons discovered him on the floor by his bed, finding it hard to breathe. They phoned everywhere they could. Only the local firemen responded. Around 10 pm F was driven off by the firemen to the hospital in the nearest town where he died at 5 am. He spent the last few hours of his long life, precipitously removed from his home, with sparse medical attention. Under the circumstances, for which nobody involved was to blame, he died arbitrarily separated from all that body of human experience, learnt over centuries, concerning the task of being with, and accompanying, the dying.

When he was young there were few doctors in this alpine region and people were accustomed to coping with illness (and dying) amongst themselves. By the time the sons were born there was a national medical service; doctors answered calls in the middle of the night and came to the house, hospitals were enlarged. The villagers gradually became dependent upon a professional medical practice and took few decisions themselves. Ten years ago with privatisation and deregulation, things changed again. Today medical care in an emergency has been reduced to a service of enforced transport. F died nowhere.

Ways of Dying

Iona Heath

Ways of Dying

Society, art, culture, the whole of human civilization is nothing but evasion, one great collective self-delusion, the intention of which is to make us forget that all the time we are falling through the air, at every moment getting closer to death.

SVEN LINDQVIST[1]

Contents

1 INTRODUCTION

I write to find my way. My signposts are words – those of my patients and my friends, and those of writers whose extraordinary talents teach us how words work and about their capacity to hold and communicate meaning and to make us feel less alone. My method is defended by Walter Benjamin:

> Learning was a form of collecting, as in the quotations and excerpts from daily reading which Benjamin accumulated in notebooks that he carried everywhere and from which he would read aloud to his friends. Thinking was also a form of collecting, at least in its preliminary stages. He conscientiously logged stray ideas; developed mini-ideas in letters to friends.[2]

More recently, complexity theory lends support with the notion that new meaning emerges from chaos.[3]

The great 19th century Russian radical Alexander Herzen included within his autobiography a chapter rather cumbersomely entitled 'A relevant chrestomathy from the later years'.[4] This strange word combines the Greek words for useful and learning and it is used to describe a collection of short quotations, especially one that is compiled to help in the learning of a language. In a sense, what follows is my personal annotated chrestomathy for a language of dying which makes sense in the context of my work as a general practitioner over many years. It describes a journey within which the words of poets, writers and thinkers illuminate the struggles of ordinary people and the details of lives and deaths which are always in some measure extraordinary.

Fifty-six million people die each year. Even if each death affects only five other people, the total number affected each year approaches 300 million or 5% of the world's population.[5] Dying permeates living, and yet much of the public response to death and dying remains polarised between sensationalism and silence.

NOTES AND REFERENCES

1 Lindqvist S. *Exterminate All the Brutes.* London: Granta Books, 1997, p. 95.

2 Sontag S. *Under the Sign of Saturn.* London: Vintage, 1996, p. 127.

3 Sweeney K. *Complexity in Primary Care: understanding its value.* Oxford: Radcliffe Publishing, 2006.

4 Herzen A. *My Past and Thoughts* (1913). Berkeley: University of California Press, 1999, p. 643.

5 Singer PA and Bowman KW. Quality care at the end of life. *British Medical Journal.* 2002; **324**: 1291–2.

2 THE DENIAL OF DEATH

Some years ago, an elderly patient on my list was admitted to hospital when the warden in her sheltered accommodation called an ambulance after she collapsed. She was in her late 80s, a widow and very frail. A furore over ageism in medicine was at its height and, perhaps as a result, she was admitted to a coronary care unit and received the highest possible standard of care, including fibrinolytic treatment delivered according to the latest evidence-based guidelines. She made a good recovery and was discharged home, apparently well, a week later. I went to see her and found her to be very grateful for the care that she had been given but profoundly shocked by a course of treatment that she perceived to be completely inappropriate. She explained to me that not only her husband but almost all of her generation of friends and acquaintances were already dead, that her physical frailty prevented her doing almost all the things that she had previously enjoyed and that she had no desire to live much longer. No-one had asked her about any of this or attempted to discover whether the effective and therefore recommended treatment for her condition was appropriate in her particular case.[1] She died three weeks later while asleep in bed. The considerable costs of her earlier treatment had been futile, distressing and wasteful.

As a general practitioner I am conscious of failing many of my patients – none more so than those who are dying. Why is it that so few of our patients die what would be recognised or described as a good death? What indeed is a good death? What manner of dying do we want for ourselves and those we love? Talking to friends and colleagues, I discover that many are able to describe their involvement in a particularly special death, where the dying person seemed able to control and orchestrate the process and to die with a dignity and calm that left everyone around them, the doctor included, feeling privileged to have been part of the story, and in some strange way enriched by it. But what is striking is how rare these deaths are. So many more are bungled and undignified, marked by overwhelming fear or suffering or both, and leaving those remaining, again including the doctor, with feelings of anger, guilt and sorrow. What goes wrong?

In *A Fortunate Man*, John Berger emphasised the centrality of the role of the general practitioner in relation to death.

The doctor is the familiar of death. When we call for a doctor, we are asking him to cure us and to relieve our suffering, but, if he cannot cure us, we are also asking him to witness our dying. The value of the witness is that he has seen so many others die . . . He is the living intermediary between us and the multitudinous dead. He belongs to us and he has belonged to them. And the hard but real comfort which they offer through him is still that of fraternity.[2]

However, during the last 100 years, the spectacular success of scientific medicine has allowed doctors to turn away from this traditional role as the 'familiar of death'. The technological challenge of prolonging life has gradually taken priority over the quality of the life lived. By dangerous and insidious processes, we have lost sight of the extent to which how we live matters more than when we die. Perversely, nowhere is this more clear than in the care of the dying.

The hubris of scientific medicine fuels ever-increasing public expectations of perfect health and consistent longevity, and these processes are eagerly exploited by both journalists and politicians, and, most of all, by the pharmaceutical industry. The aim of health care and the endpoint against which it is evaluated has become, to a very great extent, the simple prolongation of life. We talk all the time about preventable deaths – as if death could ever be prevented rather than postponed.[3] We indulge in activities and restraints that we suppose will make us live longer,[4] and the timeliness of many deaths seems never to be discussed.

Standards of health care are dictated more and more by evidence-based protocols which, by their nature, regard patients as standardised units of disease. Such protocols have no way of accommodating the unique story of the individual – the particular values, aspirations and priorities of each different person and the way that these shift over time. As a direct result, a rational evidence-based intervention of proven efficacy can turn out to be inappropriate, wasteful and futile

Western societies collude in what Philip Larkin described as 'the costly aversion of the eyes from death'.[5] The cost is monetary, but it is also one which takes a deep toll of our experience of both living and dying. Despite the expensive pretensions of medicine, death remains the inevitable end of life, and is often unpredictable, arbitrary and unjust; yet it is seen more and more as a simple failure of medicine and doctors. Medicine cannot promise the relief of all bodily discomfort and pain, yet we become ever less tolerant of these and ever more convinced that we have a right to perfect health. Scientists and doctors, but also journalists and politicians, carry a great responsibility for perpetuating these dangerous illusions, which serve to further damage, demoralise, stigmatise and disappoint the dying and those suffering from chronic diseases that can be treated but not cured.

The continuing emphasis on lifestyle risk factors for disease creates a climate of victim blaming which adds a sense of guilt to the distress and terror suffered by those arbitrarily afflicted by serious disease. Susan Sontag notes that, in the films of Ingmar Bergman, the realm of justice – the notion that characters get what they 'deserve' – is rigorously excluded.[6] This may explain the bleakness of some of the films but it is also underpins their power and their authenticity. We all try to make sense of our lives by constructing a coherent narrative that includes notions of cause and effect. We tell ourselves and each other that something happened because we did this or because that was done to us, but the link between cause and effect is often much more tenuous than we like to imagine.[7] The current wave of exaggerated claims for the power of preventive medicine is part of the same phenomenon.[8] We want to believe that if we behave well, eat the right foods in moderation, exercise regularly and so on, we will be rewarded with a long and healthy life. But as Ingmar Bergman seeks to show us, it is not necessarily so. Arthur Kleinman reminds us that:

> Cancer is an unsettling reminder of the obdurate grain of unpredictability and uncertainty and injustice – value questions, all – in the human condition.[9]

The contemporary denial of death imposes additional burdens on both patients and doctors. Feeling themselves blamed for every death, doctors are driven by a sense of guilt and unease to struggle more and more for the prolongation of life, often at the expense of its quality. A study of the care of patients with either advanced cancer or advanced dementia, dying in an acute hospital in the US, revealed that for 24% of both groups cardiopulmonary resuscitation was attempted, and 55% of those with dementia died with feeding tubes in place.[10] The effect is that 'it is now almost impossible to die with dignity in the USA unless one is poverty stricken'.[11]

> One of the most ill-starred meetings in modern medicine is that between a frail, defenceless old man nearing the end of his life, and an agile young intern at the beginning of his career.[12]

Murray and colleagues have used qualitative research techniques to compare the experience of dying in richer and poorer countries, and have found that while patients in Kenya describe their desire to die in order to be free of pain, patients in Scotland describe wanting to die because of the side-effects of medical treatment.[13] This seems a terrible indictment of modern medical care.

Christopher Ricks has described Samuel Beckett as:

> . . . the great writer of an age which has created new possibilities and impossibilities even in the matter of death. Of an age which has dilated longevity, until it is as much a nightmare as a blessing.[14]

It seems that ordinary people are more and more aware of the nightmare, particularly as they grow older, and have made clear that awareness through their enthusiastic adoption of advance directives and living wills.

I have argued that the hubris and ambition of biomedical science is largely responsible for the dangerous and damaging denial of death within contemporary society. However, visiting Daniel Libeskind's new building for the Jewish Museum in Berlin and standing in the cold empty darkness of the Holocaust Tower, I began to wonder whether the genocidal ugliness of so much death in the most recently completed century was at least partly responsible for our aversion; whether the causes might be as much cultural as scientific.

NOTES AND REFERENCES

1 Misselbrook D. *Thinking about Patients.* Newbury: Petroc Press, 2001, p. 41.

2 Berger J and Mohr J. *A Fortunate Man.* Harmondsworth: Allen Lane, The Penguin Press, 1967, p. 68.

3 Fitzpatrick M. *The Tyranny of Health: doctors and the regulation of lifestyle.* London: Routledge, 2001, p. 3.

4 Thomas L. *The Fragile Species.* New York: Scribner, 1992.
'Dieting, jogging, and thinking different thoughts may make us feel better while we are in good health, but they will not change the incidence or outcome of most of our real calamities.'

5 Larkin P. Wants. In: *Collected Poems.* London: Faber and Faber, 1988, p. 42.

6 Sontag S. Persona. *Sight and Sound.* 1967; 36(4): 186–91.

7 Miller G. Linked: a landmark in sound, an invisible artwork, a walk. 2003. www. linkedM11.info (accessed 5 October 2006). 'Events happen, then slip away while stories step into their place. On second telling our accounts start to re-shape themselves according to their own needs. Eventually a tale re-told will completely covers the event that gave it life, obscuring complexities, tidying contradictions, playing for laughs or tears.'

8 Sackett DL. The arrogance of preventive medicine. *Canadian Medical Association Journal.* 2002; 167: 363–4.

9 Kleinman A. *The Illness Narratives: suffering, healing and the human condition.* New York: Basic Books, 1988, p. 20.

10 Ahronheim JC, Morrison RS, Baskin SA, Morris J and Meier DE. Treatment of the dying in the acute care hospital. Advanced dementia and metastatic cancer. *Archives of Internal Medicine* 1996; 156: 2094–100.

11 Ricks C. *Beckett's Dying Words. The Clarendon Lectures 1990.* Oxford: Oxford University Press, 1995, p. 41.

12 Keizer B. My father's death. In: Bamforth I (ed) *The Body in the Library: a literary anthology of modern medicine.* London: Verso, 2003, p. 388.

13 Murray SA, Grant E, Grant A and Kendall M. Dying from cancer in developed and

developing countries: lessons from two qualitative interview studies of patients and their carers. *British Medical Journal.* 2003; **326**: 368–71.

14 Ricks C. *Beckett's Dying Words. The Clarendon Lectures 1990.* Oxford: Oxford University Press, 1995, p. 33.

3 THE GIFT OF DEATH

Contemporary society seems to have lost all sense of the value of death; of the indissoluble linking of death to life; of death as integral to life. The 17th century physician, Sir Thomas Browne was very clear that:

> . . . we are happier with death than we should have been without it.[1]

Paradoxically, it is death that gives us time and its passing, without which we would be lost in a welter of eternity with no reason ever to act or, indeed, to live.

On 1 August 1400, Margherita, the wife of the Bohemian humanist Johannes von Saaz, died in childbirth. The following day, von Saaz began to write his masterpiece, the play *Death and the Ploughman*, which he himself described as an attack on the inevitability of death.[2] The play presents a conversation between death and a ploughman whose loved wife has just died. Within the repetitive ruminations of his grieving, the ploughman rails against death:

> Butcher most wrathful of all creatures; killer most terrible of all peoples, vengeful destroyer of flesh, death, be thou cursed.

In response, Death calmly and systematically argues Sir Thomas Browne's position:

> Reflect for a moment, in your vanity and folly; delve in the poor soil of your reason and you will uncover the truth: if, since the first man was expressed out of clay, if we had not harvested men from the earth, animals from the wastes and wilds, fish from the waters of the deep, the very air would be thick with flies, and none could withstand them.
>
> . . .
>
> You have seen nothing of the workings of nature; you have understood nothing of the way things grow out of each other; you know nothing of how the world works by transformation and decay . . .

Without death, there is no time, no growth, no change.

In his poem, *Mr Cogito and Longevity*, Zbigniev Herbert writes of his fear of immortality. Mr Cogito is Herbert's alter ego:

> to the end
> Mr Cogito would like to sing
> the beauty of the passage of time
>
> this is why he doesn't gulp down Geleé Royale
> or drink elixirs
> doesn't make a pact with Mephisto
> with the care of a good gardener
> he cultivates the wrinkles on his face
> humbly accepts calcium
> deposited in his veins
> he is delighted by lapses of memory
> he was tormented by memory
> immortality
> since childhood
> put him in a state
> of trembling fear
> why should the gods be envied?
>
> – for celestial draughts
> – for a botched administration
> – for unsatiated lust
>
> – for a tremendous yawn[3]

Death is resented and feared because it brings an end to human joy, but it also brings an end to fear and pain and suffering:

> Time is the mercy of Eternity; without Time's swiftness
> Which is the swiftest of all things: all were eternal torment.[4]

And, as Christopher Ricks adds:

> Death is, among other things, the mercy of time . . .[5]

It is no coincidence that the contemporary denial of death has been accompanied by a valuing of the length of a life over its intensity.[6] If we avert our eyes from death, we also erode the delight of living. The less we sense death, the less we live.

> Society, art, culture, the whole of human civilization is nothing but evasion, one great collective self-delusion, the intention of which is to make us forget that all the time we are falling through the air, at every moment getting closer to death.
>
> . . .
>
> The shortness of life should not paralyze us, but stop us from diluted, unconcentrated living. The task of death is to force man into essentials.[7]

Conversely a life lived to the full seems to make dying easier.

> You mustn't be horrified. This isn't a house of mourning. There are torments and physical humiliations, and some impatience because death takes its time. But we're not grieving. We've lived close to each other for almost fifty years. I was twenty-one when we were married. Should it come about that we were able to see each other again after death, if such a mysterious possibility exists, then all these . . . externals would probably be easier to bear. And death would be a relief, as Jacob would be released from his torments and I from a burdensome waiting. But death is death. No mysteries or beautiful secrets. Do you know, for that matter, what's so remarkable, a consoling thought that comes to me when I'm tormented by distress? Well, the separation would be much more painful if our marriage had not been good. We've been allowed to live with joy . . .[8]

The central human endeavour is to find meaning in life and to construct a coherent life story which makes sense of experience. Walter Benjamin wrote that:

> The amount of meaning is in exact proportion to the presence of death and the power of decay[9]

and described:

. . . the dead occurrences of the past which are euphemistically known as experience.

The processes by which we have lost sight of the importance and value of death have, in a similar way, transformed suicide from a human right into a preventable disease. Suicide is now held to be the fault of doctors in general and mental health doctors in particular. Undoubtedly, some suicide can be prevented by psychiatric care and, almost certainly, more by the more equitable distribution of hope and opportunity within society, but nonetheless suicide remains a human right. More than three centuries ago, Sir Thomas Browne understood that:

> . . . we are in the power of no calamity while death is in our own.[10]

The chemist and writer, Primo Levi, touched the limits of his strength and endurance in his determination to survive the nadir of human cruelty in Auschwitz. In 1987, he fell to his death. In *If This is a Man* he explained, with beautiful clarity, one of the great gifts of death: it may curtail our joys but it also sets limits to our misery.

> Sooner or later in life everyone discovers that perfect happiness is unrealizable, but there are few who consider the antithesis: that perfect unhappiness is equally unattainable. The obstacles preventing the realization of both these extreme states are of the same nature: they derive from our human condition which is opposed to everything infinite. Our ever-insufficient knowledge of the future opposes it: and this is called, in the one instance, hope, and in the other, uncertainty of the following day. The certainty of death opposes it: for it places a limit on every joy, but also on every grief. The inevitable material cares oppose it: for as they poison every lasting happiness, they equally assiduously distract us from our misfortunes and make our consciousness of them intermittent and hence supportable.[11]

Most people most of the time want to live forever, but most people some of the time and some people most of the time do not. As Samuel Beckett puts it:

> Better on your arse than on your feet,
> Flat on your back than either, dead than the lot.[12]

And in *Malone Dies*, Beckett seems to echo Sir Thomas Browne in finding happiness in the inevitability of death:

> To know you can do better next time, unrecognizably better, and that there is no next time, and that it is a blessing there is not, there is a thought to be going on with.[13]

NOTES AND REFERENCES

1 Browne T. Religio Medici I.44. 1643. In: Claire Preston (ed) *Sir Thomas Browne: selected writings*. Manchester: Carcanet Press Limited, 1995, p. 22.

2 von Saaz J. *Death and the Ploughman*. Translated by Michael West. London: Methuen Drama, 2002.

3 Herbert Z. Mr Cogito and Longevity. *Report from the Besieged City and Other Poems*. Oxford: Oxford University Press, 1987, pp. 24–5. Reprinted by permission of Oxford University Press.

4 William Blake. *Milton: a poem in two books, to justify the ways of god to men* (1804). Reproduced by Tate Gallery Publications for the William Blake Trust, 1993, p. 73.

5 Ricks C. *Beckett's Dying Words. The Clarendon Lectures 1990*. Oxford: Oxford University Press, 1995, p. 24.

6 Skrabanek P. *The Death of Humane Medicine and the Rise of Coercive Healthism*. London: The Social Affairs Unit, 1994.

7 Lindqvist S. *Exterminate All the Brutes*. London: Granta Books, 1998, p. 95.

8 Bergman I. *Private Confessions*. London: The Harvill Press, 1996, pp. 98–9.

9 Sontag S. *Under the Sign of Saturn*. London: Vintage, 1996, pp. 125–6.

10 Browne T. Religio Medici I.44. 1643. In: Claire Preston (ed) *Sir Thomas Browne: selected writings*. Manchester: Carcanet Press Limited, 1995, p. 22.

11 Levi P. *If This is a Man* (1958). London: Sphere Books, 1987, p. 23.

12 Beckett S. *Collected Poems in English and French*. New York: Grove Press, 1977, p. 127. Reprinted by permission of Grove/Atlantic Inc, New York.

13 Beckett S. *Malone Dies* (1951). London: Penguin Books, 1962, p. 101.

4 WAYS OF DYING

One can die but once, but there are many manners of death.[1]

My mother-in-law died when our children were aged six and four. We had shared the house since before they were born. After she retired, she began to lose weight and put it down to having the opportunity to do more walking. However, it was not long before she was diagnosed as having inoperable cancer of the stomach and told that she had three months to live. With an obedience that was both astonishing and quite uncharacteristic, she died three months later, to the day. She was brave and open and set about distributing gifts of money to her many friends, so that Mrs Thatcher would not get her hands on it. The children reacted quite differently to her illness. The six-year-old girl climbed into bed with her grandmother, helped her to wash and read her stories. The younger boy seemed frightened by the changes he saw and was much more diffident. Shortly after she had died, we took the children to see the film *Superman*. An early scene shows Clark Kent's father collapsing and dying of a heart attack outside in the farmyard as the rest of the family eats breakfast. Our son leaned over and in a loud whisper declared that when he died, he wanted it to be like that. He had seen and understood that sudden death is easier for the one who dies although tougher for those left behind, whereas the reverse is usually true for the slower more protracted death endured by his grandmother.

The novelist, Mary Wesley, reached a similar conclusion, although she was more optimistic about the reactions of those who loved her.

> My family has a propensity – it must be our genes – for dropping dead. Here one minute, gone the next. Neat. I pray that I have inherited this gene. I have no wish to linger, to become a bed-bound bore. A short sharp shock for my loved ones is what I want: nicer for them, lovely for me.[2]

This is a frequently expressed view but, on closer examination, it is perhaps just another manifestation of the contemporary denial of death. The belief that a sudden death is better for the one who dies is one that attaches no value to the opportunities provided by a final illness. These include the chance to leave one's affairs in order, to contribute to the planning of one's funeral, to share and relive memories, to say farewell, to give and seek forgiveness,[3] and to say the things that should be said:

> We must talk to each other as much as we can.
> When one of us dies, there will be some things the other will never
> be able to talk of with anyone else.[4]

Roberto Juarroz, the great Argentinean poet, seems to express the same feeling:

> I am looking at a tree
> You are looking at something else in the distance
> But I know that if I don't look at this tree
> You will look at it for me
> And you know that if you don't look at what you are looking at
> I will look at it for you.
> It's no longer enough for each of us
> To look with the other
> We've got to where, if one of us
> Isn't there, the other will look
> At what has to be looked at.
> All that remains for us to do now
> Is to establish a look
> That will look at what
> We both have to look at
> When both of us are no longer anywhere.[5]

Dying gives us an opportunity to make life whole. A sudden death is oddly unfinished and it is perhaps this sense of incompleteness that adds to the distress of those who are left. I hope, in time, to persuade our son to reconsider his position.

In his poem *The Dead*,[6] Miroslav Holub also writes about different ways of dying:

> After the third operation, his heart
> pierced like an old carnival target,
> he woke in his bed and said,
> 'Now I'll be fine,
> like a sunflower, and by the way

have you ever seen horses make love?'
He died that night.
And another plodded on for eight
milk and water years
like a long-haired waterplant
in a sour creek,
as if he stuck his pale face out
on a skewer from behind the graveyard wall.
Finally his face disappeared.
In both cases the angel of death
stamped his hob-nailed boot
on their medulla oblongata.
I know they died the same death
but I don't think they died
in the same way.

At first sight, Holub seems to be arguing in favour of a sudden death, but the first protagonist is already sick and this seems more an argument about the need to live to the limit and to wear out our health rather than to nurse our lives out to the longest possible length.[7] It is another plea for prioritising the manner of our living over its duration.

Dying is an integral part of living and part of the story of a life. It is the last chance to find meaning and to make coherent sense of what has gone before.

> Illness story making and telling are particularly prevalent among the elderly. They frequently weave illness experience into the apparently seamless plot of their life stories, whose denouement they are constantly revising. In the terminal phase of life, looking backward constitutes much of the present. That gaze back over life's difficult treks is as fundamental to this ultimate stage of the life cycle as dream making is in adolescence and young adulthood . . . Illness, assimilated to a life story, helps the elderly patient illustrate life's high and low points . . . For the care giver what is important is to witness a life story, to validate its interpretation, and to affirm its value.[8]

Finding meaning in the story of a life is an act of creation.

The story of our life is never an autobiography, always a novel . . . Our memories are just another artifice . . .[9]

An autobiographical fact can be pure fiction. And no less reliable for that.[10]

Meaning is constructed from memory and imagination, from the form of knowing that was described by the 17th century Neapolitan thinker Giambatista Vico, and which is different from knowing that or knowing how.

> . . . the central principle which is Vico's ultimate claim to immortality: the principle according to which man can understand himself because, and in the process, of understanding his past – because he is able to reconstruct imaginatively (in Aristotle's phrase) what he did and what he suffered, his hopes, wishes, fears, efforts, his acts and his works, both his own and those of his fellows.[11]

Every day, each of us selects, and makes explicit, perceptions from the myriad of sensations, thoughts and feelings that are experienced. These perceptions become fixed in memory and are used to create a story of that day and, cumulatively, the story of a life.

> To know and not to speak.
> In that way one forgets.
> What is pronounced strengthens itself.
> What is not pronounced tends to non-existence.[12]

Coherence, dignity and meaning within the accumulated story make it possible for the protagonist to die with a sense of worth and achievement, and this perhaps explains the significance of retelling and reliving important events at the end of life and the very real comfort that can be realised for both the dying person and those who will be left behind by talking through past events and looking again at shared photographs. Relatives and friends can continue the narrative even after the person is too weak to contribute, and in so doing give comfort to everyone.

> Truth grows gradually in us, like a musician who plays a piece again and again until he hears it for the first time.[13]

What we need perhaps is a secular version of shriving – the old ritual of hearing confession, imposing a penance and granting absolution. This could provide the opportunity to review a life and to make an account; to salve bad memories and allow for expressions of remorse and forgiveness. The giving of short shrift, cutting off any sense of the wholeness of a life, has become endemic, and both living and dying are the poorer for it.

NOTES AND REFERENCES

1 Conrad J. *Victory* (1915). London: Penguin Books, 1963, p. 283.

2 Quoted in *The Time of Your Life: getting on with getting on*. Compiled by John Burningham. London: Bloomsbury Publishing, 2003.

3 Tolstoy L. *War and Peace* (1865–1869). Glasgow: The University Press, 1938, Vol 6, p. 122.
'When two people quarrel they are always both in fault, and one's own guilt suddenly becomes terribly serious when the other is no longer alive.'

4 Attributed to both Matisse and Picasso by Françoise Gilot. Quoted in the Matisse Picasso exhibition at Tate Modern, 11 May to 18 August 2002. www.tate.org.uk/modern/exhibitions/matissepicasso/room14.htm (accessed 5 October 2006).

5 Juarroz R. From *Poésie verticale (I à IV)*. Brussels: Talus d'approche, 1996. Translated from the French by John Berger.

6 Holub M. *Interferon, or On Theater*. Oberlin: Oberlin College Press, 1982. Reprinted by permission of Oberlin College Press.

7 Shapin S and Martyn C. How to live forever: lessons of history. *British Medical Journal*. 2000; **321**: 1580–2.

8 Kleinman A. *The Illness Narratives: suffering, healing and the human condition*. New York: Basic Books, 1988, pp. 49–50.

9 Barnes J. *Love etc.* London: Jonathan Cape, 2000, p. 13.

10 Brian Friel, quoted in: O'Toole F. Programme note for Brian Friel's *Faith Healer*. Almeida Theatre Company, 2001, London.

11 Berlin I. Vico's concept of knowledge. In: Berlin I. *Against the Current. Essays in the history of ideas* (1955). London: Pimlico, 1997, p. 114.

12 Miłosz C. Reading the Japanese Poet Issa (1762–1826) (1978). In: *New and Collected Poems 1931–2001*. London: Penguin Classics, 2005, p. 350.

13 Michaels A. *Fugitive Pieces*. London: Bloomsbury Publishing, 1998, p. 251.

5 ALIVE UNTIL DEAD

Dying is part of life and not part of death: dying must be lived. Samuel Beckett's Malone understands this very clearly:

> All I ask is that the last of mine, as long as it lasts, should have living for its theme, that is all, I know what I mean. If it begins to run short of life I shall feel it.[1]

Alexander Herzen believed that the ultimate goal of life was life itself, 'that the day and the hour were ends in themselves, not a means to another day or another experience'.[2] This valuing of the experiences of the immediate present provides the stuff of life and ensures the living within dying. A dying friend, even when overcome with fatigue and weakness, talked of 'the possibility of pleasure in the smallest of things – even in a fleeting thought'. Byron believed that the goal of life was sensation:

> The great object in life is Sensation – to feel that we exist, even though in pain; it is this 'craving void' which drives us to gaming, to battle, to travel, to intemperate but keenly felt pursuits of every description whose principal attraction is the agitation inseparable from their accomplishment.[3]

The dying patients in the East End of London who spoke to the sociologist Michael Young expressed much the same view, challenging conventional approaches to the problem of pain at the end of life:

> You need pain so you are aware you are alive. Everyone says 'do you have any pain?' anxiously. It should be the other way round.
>
> Julia Searle (aged 54 years)[4]

While recognising that the ability to control pain is fundamental to the care and comfort of dying patients, Young understood that:

> Once they had assured themselves that pain was controllable – could be reduced if it got worse – they chose to tolerate it . . . Drug intake was a measuring rod. Taking less was progress, more decline. It was as if the pain

belonged to death, and if it could be managed without artificial aid, or with less, it meant that death was not so near. If this is the attitude, then the message from the hospice at St Christopher's – that cancer pain can be cut right down by opiates – is not going to penetrate all that quickly, as perhaps it should not if it reduces the measure of control that people have.

. . .

> No doctor knows how much pain you have; only you know that, and if you can vary the level and explore it, you can exercise some autonomy in a matter that is quite vital to you. The pain is almost welcome because you have the freedom to feel pain, or not, as you wish.[5]

Thus pain is not always destructive – it can be confirming.

The German philosopher Hans-Georg Gadamer died in March 2002 at the age of 102. Perhaps not surprisingly, he had thought deeply about death and dying.

> The doctor is burdened with terrible problems, especially in treating the dying. To what extent may the doctor seek to ease the patient's suffering when what is thereby taken away is not only the patient's pain but also their 'person', their freedom and responsibility for their own life, and ultimately even awareness of their own death?[6]

Biomedical technology enables doctors to relieve many of the symptoms of dying, but Gadamer argues that, in so doing, they deprive their patients of the experience of their own dying. Young's informants compared the technical relief of pain with the existential reality of facing death for which there is no biomedical response except perhaps the crude sedation of opiates and other medications.

> They have been bent lower and lower by an accumulation of distress which can be far more formidable in its totality than the sort of pain which opiates can relieve and, above all, they can fear becoming more and more dependent on their carers, losing all their independence and eventually becoming too much of a burden to bear.[7]

It is possible that, at the beginning of the 21st century, our care of the dying is at the point where obstetrics was when women were at last offered effective pain relief but before they reclaimed the right to choose whether or not they wanted it or whether they wanted to try other ways of coping and living with the pain. We use pain killers and relieve a lot of suffering, but we anaesthetise people so that they do not feel death and so have no way of making sense of it and, in so doing, perhaps we devalue the life which is so inextricably bound to it. A 'medical' death becomes almost as truncated as a violent one. In *War and Peace*, Tolstoy describes death and dying in a time before modern pharmacology, and he also explores systematically the inverse relationship between free will and inevitability. It may be that by using pain killers and sedation we suffocate any possibility of freedom in death, and so emphasise only its inevitability.

NOTES AND REFERENCES

1 Beckett S. *Malone Dies* (1951). London: Penguin Books, 1962, p. 29.

2 Berlin I. Herzen and his memoirs. In: Berlin I. *Against the Current. Essays in the history of ideas* (1955). London: Pimlico, 1997, p. 211.

3 George Gordon Noel Byron (1788–1824), British poet, letter, 6 September 1813, written to Annabella Millbanke, later Lady Byron. In: Leslie A Marchand (ed) *Byron's Letters and Journals*, vol 3, Cambridge, MA: Harvard University Press, 1974.

4 Young M and Cullen L. *A Good Death: conversations with East Londoners*. London: Routledge, 1996, p. 132.

5 Ibid, p. 130.

6 Gadamer H-G. *The Enigma of Health*. Palo Alto: Stanford University Press, 1996, p. 172.

7 Young M and Cullen L. *A Good Death: conversations with East Londoners*. London: Routledge, 1996, p. 138.

6 HOW IS IT POSSIBLE TO DIE?

It is difficult to die. The transition from a strong healthy body to one capable of slipping gently away into death is hard. Unless it is the result of sudden and overwhelming catastrophe, the transition cannot be achieved without experiencing fatigue and weakness and other physical symptoms of debility and decline. The ambition that medical care should enable people to die 'symptom-free'[1] seems to me an unattainable and dangerously dishonest chimera.[2]

By implying that dying can be detached from suffering, medicine makes a false promise and devalues, as somehow obsolete and unnecessary, the age-old human endeavour of facing pain and suffering with fortitude and stoicism.[3] This seems a very serious error.

Will, desire and aspiration are all frustrated by the body's betrayal, and yet strength must be found to reconcile mind and imagination to the finality, irreversibility and loneliness of death.

Yes, there is no good pretending, it is hard to leave everything.[4]

Life is finite, but the feelings and thoughts provoked by it seem infinite. Each of us is able to imagine the sun rising on the day after our own funeral. This ability to project ourselves into an imagined future fuels a continuing sense of hope.

. . . man's very ability to envisage his own future lends to it such a tangible presence that he cannot grasp the thought of its actually coming to an end. We can be said to have a future for as long as we are not aware that we have no future. The repression of death reflects the will of life.[5]

Living always has a future, even while dying, and it is important that hope, however constrained and limited, is nurtured.

Hope is itself a species of happiness, and, perhaps, the chief happiness which this world affords: but, like all other pleasures immoderately enjoyed, the excesses of hope must be expiated by pain; and expectations improperly indulged must end in disappointment.[6]

As Johnson warns, there is a delicate balance to be struck between the ultimately painful deceit of false hope and the genuine hope, albeit confined to a very limited present, of a better moment, a sunny day, a birthday or a loving contact.

There is something extraordinary about the way the human mind and spirit adapt to the slow erosion of the body by ageing or disease, constantly adjusting to altered circumstance but remaining largely unchanged with undiminished aspirations and hopes.

> I was seven, or seventeen, and I didn't know
> how ageing works, like Zeno's paradox,
> adjusting all the time, to right itself;
> yet sometimes, on a winter afternoon,
>
> I thought of someone skilled – a juggler, say –
> adapting to the pull of gravity
> by shifts and starts, till something in the flesh
> – a weightedness, a plumb-line to the earth –
> revealed itself, consenting to be still.[7]

This adaptation is part of the enduring presence of hope and a part that can be nurtured throughout a final illness.

> . . . the brilliance with which the mind makes and remakes expectations in such a way that life remains worth living . . .[8]

Gadamer invites us to believe that the final act of dying, like that of falling asleep will always evade direct experience.

> . . . there is sleep and the process of falling asleep, which are marked by a particular mysterious and obscure character which borders on that of death itself. For no one can 'experience' their own falling asleep. What is contained in this constellation of sleep and death, of sinking into sleep and waking up again?[9]

> How is it that waking and sleeping, and life and death, represent an indissoluble unity and are connected to one another without any intermediate stage between them?[10]

The fatigue and sleepiness of a final illness can seem like a rehearsal for death.

My patients have shown me that, in dying, the time of the body and the time of the mind can very easily become disconnected. Some patients have bodies that fail well before the mind is ready to die, which exacerbates fear and anger. Others are reconciled and ready in their minds to die, long before the body is capable of dying.

> And there comes the hour when nothing more can happen and nobody more can come and all is ended but the waiting that knows itself in vain.[11]

At its worst, this predicament can lead to suicide or requests for euthanasia. It seems to me that one of the tasks of medical care is to try and bring the two times into as close a harmony as possible and that pain and suffering have an essential part to play in this process. It is clearly essential not to romanticise pain, but it is possible that pain is not the unmitigated evil dictated by the conventions of palliative care. Could it be that the presence of pain reduces frustration and anger because pain and suffering, in some way, help the sufferer to become reconciled to death?

It seems that all the things that we fight against – illness, pain and ageing – are, in some strange way, the things that make it possible to die. There seem to be parallels with pregnancy when the gradual onset of the indignities and physical discomforts of late pregnancy make the difficulties, demands and sleeplessness of looking after a tiny baby seem an improvement in life's condition. One of the things that needs to be emphasised when someone is given a fatal diagnosis is that you will not die until your body is ready to die – until it reaches the point when it actually wants to die.

> A parting gift to my body:
> just when it wishes,
> I'll breathe my last.[12]

Spinoza's theory of parallelism maintained that:

> an action in the mind is necessarily an action in the body as well, and what is a passion in the body is necessarily a passion in the mind. There is no primacy of one series over the other.[13]

This seems to suggest that the sickness of the body serves to attune the mind to the necessity of death.

> A certain readiness to perish is not so very rare, but it is seldom that you meet men whose souls, steeled in the impenetrable armour of resolution, are ready to fight a losing battle to the last, the desire of peace waxes stronger as hope declines, till at last it conquers the very desire of life.[14]

Sense making and the finding of meaning, the summation of a life within a coherent story, are processes through which the mind becomes accepting of death. Connections of love and acquaintance and relationship are crucial to this endeavour.

> The appreciation of meanings is bound within a relationship: it belongs to the sick person's spouse, child, friend, or care giver, or to the patient himself. For this reason it is usually as much hedged in with ambiguities as are those relationships themselves. But in the long, oscillating course of chronic disorder, the sick, their relatives, and those who treat them become aware that the meanings communicated by illness can amplify or dampen symptoms, exaggerate or lessen disability, impede or facilitate treatment.[15]

There is evidence to suggest that patients living in traditional communities in poorer countries have many more unmet physical needs but fewer unmet psychosocial needs than patients living in richer countries.[16] The professionalisation of palliative care and the consequent medicalisation of death seem to have deskilled and disempowered families and friends so that they are no longer able to accommodate the distress of the dying. Ways need to be found for richer countries to learn from poorer ones while, at the same time, improving the physical care of dying patients in poorer countries without damaging the very real support currently provided by family and community.

> Most other cultures, including many primitive ones whom we have subjugated to our reason and our technology, enfold their members in an art of dying as in an art of living. But we have left these awesome tasks of culture to private choice.[17]

Human lives span past, present and future. During his last illness, a friend once told me that his past seemed a failure, his future almost non-existent, and he was trapped in the misery of the present. The response must be not only to reduce the distress of the present and to attempt to locate some hope within it, but also to take an inventory of the past: to explore memory, to tell a story of achievement and to say explicitly and repeatedly all the precious things that, too often, are only said at funerals.

Doctors need to find a way of being a useful part of this necessary exploration, without intruding and without assuming understanding where there is none.

> I have had a visit. Things were going too well. I had forgotten myself, lost myself. I exaggerate. Things were not going too badly. I was elsewhere. Another was suffering. Then I had the visit. To bring me back to dying. If that amuses them. The fact is that they don't know, neither do I, but they think they know.[18]

A destructive intrusion into the delicate balance that constitutes a good dying can also be physical and more obviously medical.

> And when they cannot swallow any more someone rams a tube down their gullet, or up their rectum, and fills them full of vitaminized pap, so as not to be accused of murder.[19]

This was written more than 50 years ago. It is frightening to consider how much truer it has become over the intervening years. Medicine has not learnt when to stop.

It is very difficult to identify the moment when the pursuit of improvement in a patient's condition has become futile and it is time to switch from treatment to comfort. It is sometimes easier with cancer when patients and those who love them are often expecting deterioration, but it is much harder with those who are gently losing a battle against an accumulation of chronic diseases, especially when they are old and frail. Yet old people often help doctors by saying, if they are given the chance, that they themselves do not wish to struggle any further, but it is often harder for those who will be left behind to accept this kind of giving up. There is a great need to recast this notion of abandonment as a different sort of accompanying – a move of love and respect.

When the fatal illness appears I hope to be conscious and helped to see it clearly; the problem will be how to resist, how to avoid treatment without too much natural suffering. Disease is less frightening if one reflects on it. The endless exams, therapies, and the whole medical apparatus do not reassure me; they distress me. I will fight for power rather than calmly offer my flank to an ointment. The most urgent problem will be finding a doctor, not a cure.[20]

This deliberate detachment of the role of the doctor from the pursuit of cure frees the doctor to remake his or her relationship with the dying patient, and those around them, by focusing on the detail of present experience in the context of the particular aspirations and values of a unique life.

NOTES AND REFERENCES

1 Thomas K. *Caring for the Dying at Home: companions on the journey.* Oxford: Radcliffe Medical Press, 2003, p. 57.

2 Loeffler I. Personal view: managing chronic disease. *British Medical Journal.* 2001; **323**: 241.

3 Daniels A. Ivan Illich: 1926–2002. *The New Criterion.* 2003; **January:** 78.

4 Beckett S. *Malone Dies* (1951). London: Penguin Books, 1962, p. 130.

5 Gadamer H-G. *The Enigma of Health.* Palo Alto: Stanford University Press, 1996, p. 65.

6 Johnson S. Letter, June 8 1762. Quoted in: Boswell J. *Life of Johnson* (1791). London: Everyman's Library, 1992, pp. 232–3.

7 Burnside J. The Gravity Chair. In: *The Light Trap.* London: Jonathan Cape, 2002, p. 30. Reprinted with permission of The Random House Group Inc.

8 Young M and Cullen L. *A Good Death: conversations with East Londoners.* London: Routledge, 1996, p. 48.

9 Gadamer H-G. *The Enigma of Health.* Palo Alto: Stanford University Press, 1996, p. 131.

10 Ibid, p. 145.

11 Beckett S. *Malone Dies* (1951). London: Penguin Books, 1962, p. 84.

12 Ensei (died 1725). *Japanese Death Poems,* compiled and with an introduction by Yoel Hoffmann. Rutland, Vermont: Charles E Tuttle Company, 1996, p. 160. Reprinted by permission of Charles E Tuttle Co Inc.

13 Deleuze G. *Spinoza: practical philosophy.* San Francisco: City Lights Books, 1988, p. 18.

14 Conrad J. *Lord Jim* (1900). London: Penguin Books, 1957, p. 71.

15 Kleinman A. *The Illness Narratives: suffering, healing and the human condition.* New York: Basic Books, 1988, pp. 8–9.

16 Murray SA, Grant E, Grant A and Kendall M. Dying from cancer in developed and developing countries: lessons from two qualitative interview studies of patients and their carers. *British Medical Journal.* 2003; **326**: 368.

17 Ignatieff M. *The Needs of Strangers* (1984). London: Vintage, 1994, pp. 76–7.

18 Beckett S. *Malone Dies* (1951). London: Penguin Books, 1962, p. 118.

19 Ibid, p. 99.

20 Ceronetti G. The silence of the body. In: Bamforth I (ed) *The Body in the Library: a literary anthology of modern medicine*. London: Verso, 2003, p. 296.

7 TIME AND ETERNITY

Part of the challenge of contemporary dying is the Enlightenment legacy of the conception of time as linear and associated with a notion of progress,[1] which leaves the finitude of death in the position of a full stop and conveying a sense of failure. This linearity displaced the preceding view of time as circular, mirroring the cycles of the natural world, which more easily accommodated a place for death as an essential component of the renewal of family and community life. These shifts have been paralleled by a shifting of the location of happiness. Before the Enlightenment, happiness was primarily prospective, and people lived in hope of salvation and a joyful future. Now, happiness is almost entirely retrospective and death proportionately more dreadful. The loss of the anticipation of prospective happiness has been accompanied by a loss of connectedness and a loss of solidarity between the living and the dead.

Memory and imagination position an individual at the present moment but facing both a past and a future, each of which can be seen as a circle that closes at the present.[2]

> Man is an animal for whom Being spontaneously opens forward to the future and backwards to the past. His being is thus literally compounded of non-Being – the *Not*-yet of the future, the *No*-longer of the past. Only as he holds these two together in presence is he able to stand meaningfully in time . . .[3]

For the dying person, the circle of the past contains the story of a life but also the interconnecting stories of many other lives; and the circle of the future extends the limited life of the individual by including the continuing lives of others.

Writing about Lisbon, John Berger writes about three stages of remembering – the first memory 'displays a certain indulgence', the second 'regains control of itself' and the third 'waits to see what is going to happen next'. In this way, it is possible to understand how cycles of memory provoke the imagination of a future.[4]

Death is both the connection and the barrier between time and eternity, and this is underlined by the prevalence of doorway motifs on ancient sarcophagi and medieval tombs.[5] For some, death brings an eternity of nothingness and for others an eternity of just desserts. Both views have the capacity to offer comfort.

> My long sickness
> Of health and living now begins to mend,
> And nothing brings me all things.[6]

The notion of an eternity of just desserts in either a heaven or a hell is oddly complementary to the nature of temporal experience, employing the full extent of the human imagination to extrapolate beyond the limitations of experience towards the absolute extremes of happiness or anguish.

Other ways of looking at the connections between time and eternity can emphasise the link and make the barrier between them seem less absolute – more porous. The link is very often mediated by some kind of conception of God, however unconventional. Spinoza seemed to have a view of God as immanent within nature and the human imagination – within everything that all who live and who have ever lived hold in common – within the intensity of life itself:

> . . . the eternity of essence does not come afterwards; it is strictly con-
> temporaneous, coexistent with existence in duration . . . the good or strong
> individual is the one who exists so fully or so intensely that he has gained
> eternity in his lifetime, so that death, always extensive, always external, is
> of little significance to him. The ethical test is therefore the contrary of the
> deferred judgment . . .[7]

Boris Pasternak has a related view of God as immanent within history and human memory:

> This freedom came from the feeling that all human lives were interrelated,
> a certainty that they flowed into each other – a happy feeling that all events
> took place not only on earth, in which the dead are buried, but also in some
> other region which some called the Kingdom of God, others history, and still
> others by some other name.[8]
>
> What you don't understand is that it is possible to be an atheist, it is
> possible not to know whether God exists, or why and yet believe that man
> does not live in a state of nature but in history . . . Now what is history?

It is the centuries of systematic explorations of the riddle of death, with a view to overcoming death. That's why people discover mathematical infinity and electromagnetic waves, that's why they write symphonies. Now you can't advance in this direction without a certain faith. You can't make such discoveries without spiritual equipment.[9]

. . . he developed his old view of history as another universe, made by man with the help of time and memory in answer to the challenge of death.[10]

When his aunt is gravely ill and expected to die, the young medical student Zhivago attempts to comfort her:

You in others – this is your soul. This is what you are. This is what your consciousness has breathed and lived on and enjoyed throughout your life – your soul, your immortality, your life in others. And what now? You have always been in others and you will remain in others. And what does it matter to you if later on that is called your memory? This will be you – the you that enters the future and becomes a part of it.[11]

Seamus Heaney and George Steiner seem to agree in finding God in the achievement and scope of language. At the Memorial Service for Ted Hughes on 15 May 1999, Seamus Heaney said:

One part of Ted believed in the gene and its laws as the reality we inhabit and are bound to adjust to, since there issues from the genetic code the whole alphabet of our possibilities, from the alpha at the start of the evolutionary journey to omega at the end. But another part of him looked through the microscope and telescope into the visionary crystal, and could see Dante's eternal *margherita*, the pearl of foreverness, in the interstices of the DNA. This is the part of him that recognised that myths and fairy tales were the *poetic* code, that the body was a spirit beacon as well as a chemical formula, that it was born for both ecstasy and extinction.[12]

George Steiner finds a sense of eternity in every use of the future tense:

There is an actual sense in which every human use of the future tense of the verb 'to be' is a negation, however limited, of mortality. Even as every use of an 'if'-sentence tells of a refusal of the brute inevitability, of the despotism of the fact. 'Shall', 'will' and 'if', circling in intricate fields of semantic force around a hidden centre or nucleus of potentiality, are the passwords to hope.[13]

Reading all this, as someone who finds nothing in conventional religion, I begin to understand how the human genius for anthropomorphism generates God at the interstices of infinity and eternity, within the totality and intensity of human experience, at the limits of both memory and imagination. The Romans understood Jupiter as both the father of the gods but also as the air, Neptune as a bearded God with a trident but also as all the seas and oceans of the world.[14] The key seems to be a combination of coherence, connection and hope, all of which are essential to the doctor's conversation with those who are dying.

> Consciousness, the appetite for more and more, always more, the hunger for eternity and the thirst for infinity, the craving for God – none of these is ever satisfied. Each consciousness seeks to be itself and to be all others as well without ceasing to be itself: it seeks to be God.[15]

The vast scope and dimensions of the natural world, including those of the human body and mind, and the unpredictability and contingency of its workings, generate a desperate human need for an illusion of control. Historically, this need has been fulfilled by a notion of God, but, increasingly, since the Enlightenment, God has been displaced by science. Yet, the continuing uncertainty of human destiny demonstrates that control remains illusory and, worse, science reduces everything to number and has no way of making sense of things which have no metric and no currency of comparison, such as love, hope, trust, joy, compassion, loneliness, forgiveness and grief, all of which are crucial to finding meaning in a time of dying. Pain is perhaps another example. Science has provided us with apparently reliable ways of measuring pain with a variety of scales and scoring systems, but it remains impossible to know another's pain and to that extent pain is beyond comparison or measure.[16] In these ways, while the move from god to science has brought many benefits there have also been losses and there is a vacuum at the heart of contemporary explanation.

In his extraordinary novel *Austerlitz*, WG Sebald dissects the mysterious workings of memory and the non-linear, reverberating and resonating quality of time. In this way he reveals the porousness of the barriers between the living and the dead and between time and eternity.

> The dead are outside time, the dying and all the sick at home or in hospitals, and they are not the only ones, for a certain degree of personal misfortune is enough to cut us off from the past and the future.[17]
>
> It does not seem to me, Austerlitz added, that we understand the laws governing the return of the past, but I feel more and more as if time did not exist at all, only various spaces interlocking according to the rules of a higher form of stereometry, between which the living and the dead can move back and forth as they like, and the longer I think about it the more it seems to me that we who are still alive are unreal in the eyes of the dead, that only occasionally, in certain lights and atmospheric conditions, do we appear in their field of vision.[18]
>
> It seems to me then as if all the moments of our life occupy the same space, as if future events already existed and were only waiting for us to find our way to them at last, just as when we have accepted an invitation we duly arrive in a certain house at a given time. And might it not be . . . that we also have appointments to keep in the past, in what has gone before and is for the most part extinguished, and must go there in search of places and people who have some connection with us on the far side of time, so to speak?[19]

Many people, when acutely bereaved, and fewer people, over a longer time course, sense this porousness between dying and living, feel the presence of the dead, hear the familiar voice. Such experiences are often dismissed or ignored, but their frequency must have meaning and we need to pay more attention to their origin and significance. The pervasive lack of under-standing of these experiences adds unnecessarily to the pain and isolation of grieving.

> This last night of all, sheltered from the great wind of absence.
> The inwardness of Good-bye is tragic,
> like that of every event in which Time is manifest.[20]

Memory and imagination allow us to hold on to the dead.[21] Both are depend-ent on Giambatista Vico's form of knowing which makes possible links between cultures and individuals across and beyond time and space, because the fundamentals of what makes people human are held in common by them everywhere and at all times. This is the form of knowing that is concerned with 'motives, purposes, hopes, fears, loves and hatreds, jealousies, ambitions, outlooks and visions of reality'.[22] It is how we understand what it is to delight in the world, to fall in love, to long for someone or something, to mourn. None of the dimensions of this form of knowing can be measured, and all fall outside the scope and metric of science but Vico's understanding is nonetheless fundamental to the care of the dying.

Theatre de Complicite's magnificent play *Mnemonic*[23] explores the same form of knowing and the power of imagination to build links between human beings across extraordinary distances of time and space. The play revolves around the discovery of the body of a man, born more than 5000 years ago, buried and preserved in the ice of the Alps on the border between Austria and Italy. The text is punctuated by repeated questions which resonate across time and space and make sense in the context of any human life: 'How many mourned him when he disappeared?' 'How many songs did he know?' 'How many children did he have?' 'What word did he use to signify summer?'. These questions connect and will always connect the living and the dead.

There is much talk of the moment of death, an instant of demarcation between the living and the dead, but this very seldom tallies with the experience of those who witness dying and death.

> It is a process. People don't suddenly die. Death is not an event. Not even when they have suffered a heart attack or been in an accident, do people suddenly die. There is life long after the heart has stopped beating . . . Death is not the finite moment that we are told it is. Death is the infinite moment.[24]

Dead bodies need care and attention, and traditional rituals of care have the capacity to help both the one who has died and those left behind. I remember an old lady whose husband died during the night but who did not summon the doctor until the following morning. She explained that she had slept snuggled up to his body for 50 years and she wanted one last night. It was a form of gentle and measured leave-taking but few people today seem to have the courage and self-confidence to avail themselves of such comfort.

Seamus Heaney has described twilight as:

... that time of day when the land of the living and the land of the dead become pervious to each other, when the deserted present becomes populous with past lives ...[25]

Across the borderline of time and eternity, the dead can help the dying to die.[26]

It's the truest of all democracies, this democracy of death.[27]

Dying is a universal achievement – a test that it is impossible to fail – and there can be real comfort in thinking of those already on the other side of the borderline.

You reach a moment in life when, among the people you have known, the dead outnumber the living. And the mind refuses to accept more faces, more expressions: on every new face you encounter, it prints the old forms, for each one it finds the most suitable mask.[28]

Older people recognise this moment and it arrives earlier for doctors than for most others. After more than 30 years of working in Kentish Town in north London, my practice area is populated by generations of ghosts, waiting in half-remembered interiors alongside the changed rooms and the new inhabitants. The total population of living and dead gets denser and denser. Often the general practitioner and the dying patient share this experience and this perception.

Once people have sustained a critical number of losses – sometimes losses of health, sometimes losses of more nebulous things like dignity or reputation, but most often losses of love – it seems to become easier to die. People are more or less resilient and have greater or lesser reserves of love and health and dignity, and for some who start with very little, only one significant loss can be enough. The older one gets, the more losses one must suffer, particularly of those who are loved and loving, and when people have lost many who are important to them it becomes easier to die. The death of the others has led the way, and in this way the dead help the living to die. Perhaps it is at the moment when the dead outnumber the living that they can keep the dying company and perhaps this is why it is so much harder for the young to die.

NOTES AND REFERENCES

1 Gray J. *Al Qaeda and What it Means to be Modern.* London: Faber and Faber, 2003.

2 Berger J. Historical afterword. In: *Pig Earth* (1979). London: Chatto & Windus, 1985, p. 201.

3 Barrett W. Unamuno and the contest with death. Afterword to Unamuno M de. *The Tragic Sense of Life in Men and Nations* (1913). Princeton: Princeton University Press, 1972, p. 368.

4 Berger J and Berger Andreadakis K. The long sunset. *The Guardian*, Saturday 5 August, 2000. www.guardian.co.uk/saturday_review/story/0,,350546,00.html (accessed 5 October 2006).

5 Binski P. *Medieval Death: ritual and representation.* Ithaca: Cornell University Press, 1996.

6 Shakespeare W. *Timon of Athens.* Act 5, Scene 1.

7 Deleuze G. *Spinoza: practical philosophy.* San Francisco: City Lights Books, 1988, p. 40.

8 Pasternak B. *Doctor Zhivago* (1957). New York: Signet Books, 1960, p. 15.

9 Ibid, p. 13.

10 Ibid, p. 58.

11 Ibid, p. 60.

12 Heaney S. A Great Man and a Great Poet: address at the Memorial Service for Ted Hughes, May 13, 1999. *The Observer Review.* Sunday May 16, 1999.

13 Steiner G. *Grammars of Creation.* New Haven: Yale University Press, 2002, p. 7.

14 Berlin I. The divorce between the sciences and the humanities. In: Berlin I. *Against the Current: essays in the history of ideas.* London: Pimlico, 1979, p. 98.

15 Unamuno M de. *The Tragic Sense of Life in Men and Nations.* Princeton: Princeton University Press, 1972, p. 233.

16 Summerfied D. The invention of post-traumatic stress disorder and the social usefulness of a psychiatric category. *British Medical Journal.* 2001; **322**: 95–8.

17 Sebald WG. *Austerlitz.* London: Penguin Books, 2001, p. 143.

18 Ibid, p. 261.

19 Ibid, pp. 359–60.

20 Borges JL. To Rafael Cansinos-Asséns. In: Borges JL. *This Craft of Verse. The Charles Eliot Norton Lectures 1967–1968*. Cambridge, MA: Harvard University Press, 2000, p. 127.

21 Berger J and Trivier M. *My Beautiful*. Douchy-les-Mines: Centre Régional de la Photographie Nord Pas-de-Calais, 2004.

22 Berlin I. The divorce between the sciences and the humanities. In: Berlin I. *Against the Current: essays in the history of ideas*. London: Pimlico, 1979, p. 95.

23 Complicité. *Mnemonic*. London: Methuen, 2001.

24 Kay J. *Trumpet*. London: Picador, 1998, p. 105.

25 Heaney S. The trance and the translation. *The Guardian*, Saturday 30 November, 2002.

26 Berger J. Twelve theses on the economy of the dead. In: *Pages of the Wound: poems, drawings and photographs 1956–96*. London: Bloomsbury Publishing, 1996.

27 Tucholsky K. Apprehension. In: Bamforth I (ed) *The Body in the Library: a literary anthology of modern medicine*. London: Verso, 2003, p. 210.

28 Calvino I. *Invisible Cities* (1972). London: Vintage, 1997, p. 95.

8 WHAT THE DOCTOR NEEDS

In 2001, at the Morley Gallery in south London, there was an exhibition of Maggi Hambling's portraits of her dying father. Looking at the pictures, I found myself thinking – why does this work, how can lines of paint on a bare sheet of board be so powerful and evoke so much of what it is to love another, what it is to live, to grow old, to die? I remembered David Hockney insisting 'what the hand, the eye and the heart can do, and make, and paint, can never be replaced'.[1] Suddenly, I understood that this is the task of the doctor in the care of the dying – to use hand *and* eye *and* heart. Words are also essential, but as, inevitably, they become less accessible, touch becomes more important. Only if we use all of hand and eye and heart can we help to make possible the kind of inclusive dignity that Maggi Hambling achieves in her paintings of her father.

EYES

WG Sebald describes 'the fixed, inquiring gaze found in certain painters and philosophers who seek to penetrate the darkness which surrounds us purely by means of looking and thinking'.[2]

Doctors need eyes to see the humanity and dignity of our patients and to prevent us from turning away from suffering and distress.

> Instead of learning to look for illness in the eyes of the patient or to listen for it in the patient's voice, we try to read it off data provided by technologically sophisticated measuring instruments. Both are perhaps necessary, but it is difficult to practise both together.[3]

Once, a friend phoned me, worrying about the care that his dying friend was getting from his doctors. I knew the general practitioner well and I tried to reassure my friend that all was well. He replied: 'But the doctor and the patient do not look at each other in the eyes'. Shortly afterwards, I was talking to a dying patient of my own, I realised that I too was not looking at my patient in the eyes. I had known her for as long as I had been a general practitioner which, at the time, was 26 years. She had had a terribly hard life and for years she had worked as an early morning cleaner. Over the years, I had become aware that many doctors seemed to think that, because she was not very educated and because she had always been poor, she would accept everything that they told her. However, long before, I had learnt that all of her huge courage was built on her honesty, that she was extremely perceptive and that she could only trust those whom she believed. She needed me to look into her eyes and not to flinch but, for a few weeks, perhaps because her pain had been out of control and I had been afraid of failing her, I had been avoiding her gaze. Remembering what my friend had said, I managed to look again and it seemed better for both of us.

To look away is to reject the living person, to treat dying as part of death and not as part of life. In *Anna Karenina*, Levin finds it almost impossible to recognise, let alone acknowledge, his dying brother:

> The glittering eyes looked sternly and reproachfully at the brother as he drew near. And immediately this glance established a living relationship between living men.[4]

It is not possible to look someone in the eye and deny their humanity, but the intensity of this kind of looking is hard and, far too often, we, as doctors, flinch.

> That unwelcome flinch which the touch of egotism gives to benevolence.[5]

Perhaps we flinch because our patient is looking at us with an even greater intensity.

The earliest painted portraits that have survived were painted almost 2000 years ago. They were found at the end of the 19th century in the Egyptian province of Fayum and they were painted to be attached to the mummy of the person portrayed when he or she died. Each of the portraits has the most extraordinary eyes with a steady directness in the gaze which is almost naked in its vulnerability but, at the same time, inexplicably, conveys enormous strength.

> . . . the Fayum painter was summoned not to make a portrait . . . but to register his client, a man or a woman looking at him.[6]

John Berger writes about the way sitter and painter 'collaborated in a preparation for death'. Is this also what is required of doctor and patient? If so, how does one find the moment to start?

It was the painter rather than the 'model' who submitted to being looked at. Each portrait he made began with this act of submission.[7]

So perhaps there is a critical moment when the doctor too must submit to the gaze of the dying patient. There is no flinching in the Fayum portraits, but it is very easy to flinch, and the effect of flinching is to admit horror and to erode trust.

> Horror can go with a kind of pity. True pity is different . . . Horror is horror, even when it's small and under control and is going with pity.[8]

The required gaze is mutual, unflinching and it pays careful attention to detail, to the particular.

> One man's attitude towards another is, or should be, based on perceiving what he is in himself, uniquely, not what he has in common with all other men; only the natural sciences abstract what is common, generalise.[9]

The abstract is full of fear; the detail of the particular makes that fear manageable. Alphonse Daudet, writing in his notebooks while dying of tertiary syphilis, understood this very well:

> The doctors don't know any more than we do; in fact they know even less, because their knowledge is made up of an average drawn from observations which are generally hasty and incomplete, and because every case is a new and particular one . . . There are a great many different kinds of instrument belonging to the executioner; if they do not scare you too much, examine them carefully. It is with our torments as it is with shadows. Attention clears them up and drives them away.[10]

Looking away – flinching – is the beginning of dishonesty. A friend, coping with the diagnosis of cancer, wrote:

> What I really want as a patient is NOT more time from the doctor, nor any solution. What I want is for the doctor to remain present in the face of my fear and attempts to process the reality of my situation . . . I think that when you KNOW you're floating in massive uncertainty about life and death,

honesty really matters, because it gives you the only bearing you have (in the context of breast cancer). Otherwise it's just all hope and superstition, which don't stop you worrying at night.[11]

How is it – precisely – that some doctors and nurses are able to convey their presence and lack of flinching, while others turn away? Is it through words or touch or silence or all of these, or none, or something else – is it possible to say? The poet TS Eliot wrote that in poetry 'honesty never exists without great technical accomplishment'.[12] The same seems true in medicine.

WORDS

We need words to try and minimise the inevitable loneliness of dying, words to hold the other with us, words to make sense of shared experience.

> . . . knowing how short the time in which to say all the things that lie heavy on the heart and conscience and do all the things they have to do together, things one cannot do alone.[13]

Robert Graves described the importance of holding on to language and making use of it for as long as possible:

> Children are dumb to say how hot the day is,
> How hot the scent is of the summer rose,
> How dreadful the black wastes of evening sky,
> How dreadful the tall soldiers drumming by.
> But we have speech, to chill the angry day,
> And speech, to dull the rose's cruel scent.
> We spell away the overhanging night,
> We spell away the soldiers and the fright.
> There's a cool web of language winds us in,
> Retreat from too much joy or too much fear:
> We grow sea-green at last and coldly die
> In brininess and volubility.
> But if we let our tongues lose self-possession,
> Throwing off language and its watery clasp
> Before our death, instead of when death comes,

Facing the wide glare of the children's day,
Facing the rose, the dark sky and the drums,
We shall go mad no doubt and die that way.[14]

Language is 'social throughout its entire range and in each and every of its factors, from the sound image to the furthest reaches of abstract meaning'.[15] Words are always used to find another and to forge a connection, an understanding, with that other human individual and they come ready freighted with meaning and history. Borges described words as 'symbols for shared memories'.[16] Yet each of us, while using words, makes them anew, annexes them for our own purposes. This is the power, the adaptability and the inherent difficulty of language.

Carl Edvard Rudebeck describes the space between an inner horizon of the biology of the body and an outer horizon of the external world and our relationship with it. Within this space, symptoms are both generated and explained.[17] The relationship between inner and outer is similar to that used by John Berger to understand faces:

> . . . the traces left by experience on a person's face are the traces of meetings (or struggles) between the person's inner needs or intentions and the demands or offers of the outside world. Put differently: marks of experience on a face are the lines of conjuncture between two moulds; both moulds are social products, but one contains a self and the other history.[18]

A friend, a man dying of cancer, maintained that the inner horizon of a body subjected to serious disease is even more difficult for men to confront and articulate because men tend to be more focused on the outer horizon, whereas the whole experience of menstruation and then pregnancy means that the inner horizon is somehow more accessible to women. Is this true? I am not sure but it is clear that everyone has difficulty communicating their experience of Rudebeck's inner horizon – finding and trusting the appropriate words. In this context, 'pain' is a word both essential and slippery. Pain is always located at the inner horizon; it has no objective manifestation or measure. Each person experiences pain alone and can have no direct experience of another's pain and so, to be understood, each must depend both on words to communicate their predicament and on the listener's imagination, the listener's capacity for Vico's form of imaginative knowing.

Any utterance occurs within the history of a particular dialogue, and this historical context of an utterance about anything, but perhaps particularly about pain, refracts, adds to, or subtracts the amount and kind of meaning. The nature of the relationship between speaker and listener determines how much can be communicated. This underlies the importance of a continuing relationship between a particular doctor and a dying patient. Tragically, current political aspirations for medicine in general, and general practice in particular, do not value continuity of care, prioritise technical expertise and cling to the model of the body as a machine. This context serves to minimise medicine's perception of suffering, and colludes in a denial of death. A proper engagement with suffering and appropriate care of the dying demand continuity of care and an ongoing commitment between two named individuals.

In his Nobel lecture in 1980, Czesław Miłosz described 'two attributes of the poet: avidity of the eye and the desire to describe that which he sees'.[19] This linking of eyes and words makes very clear the relevance of poetry to the work of doctors and perhaps particularly in the care of those who are dying. The poet's example of the very careful translation into words of what is seen sets a standard of intensity to which doctors must aspire. Bakhtin points out that the words of poetry have particular significance because they have the power to extend beyond individual human lives towards eternity.

> Of course, even the poetic word is social, but poetic forms reflect lengthier social processes . . . requiring centuries to unfold.[20]

Poetry can have the quality of touch despite separation in both time and space.

> And when it comes, one feels the touch of poetry, that particular tingling of poetry.[21]

By exploring what is held in common, poetry connects past, present and future lives, and this sense of connection and meaning is an essential component of a peaceful dying.

Terror of the unknown and the uncontrollable is never far away and loneliness and fear are, as always, most overwhelming at night.

Waking at four to soundless dark, I stare.
In time the curtain-edges will grow light.
Till then I see what's really always there:
Unresting death, a whole day nearer now,
Making all thought impossible but how
And where and when I shall myself die.
Arid interrogation: yet the dread
Of dying, and being dead,
Flashes afresh to hold and horrify.[22]

Discomfiting memories are always worst at night, and when the possibility of imagining a better future is cut off, the dissatisfactions of the past and the misery of the present loom ever larger.

> . . . he was having many difficult sensations, innumerable impressions of winter, winters of seven decades superimposed . . . And none of this was clearly communicable, nor indeed worth communicating. It was simply part of the continuing life of every human being. Everybody was filled with visions that had been repressed, and amassed involuntarily, and when you were sick they were harder to disperse.[23]

> Flayed alive by memory, his mind crawling with cobras, not daring to dream or think and powerless not to, his cries were of two kinds, those having no other cause than moral anguish and those, similar in every respect, by means of which he hoped to forestall same.[24]

We can pay healing attention to fear only if we can locate it and, as doctors, we can discover it only by inviting words, by listening and by carefully and deliberately imagining. Beckett's Malone mocks his fears to keep them at bay, but the fear of the loss of dignity and control involved in both death throes and a death rattle is palpable.

> Throes are the only trouble, I must be on my guard against throes.[25]

> And the rattle, what about the rattle? Perhaps it is not *de rigueur* after all. To have vagitated and not be bloody well able to rattle. How life dulls the power of protest to be sure.[26]

Perhaps every dying person lives with fears of throes and rattles but they are very seldom spoken. Perhaps, we should encourage those we care for to follow Philip Larkin's example and that of Beckett's Malone, and write down the fears that come in the middle of the night so that they can be examined together in the light of day.

> I did not want to write, but I had to resign myself to it in the end. It is in order to know where I have got to, where he has got to. At first I did not write, I just said the thing. Then I forgot what I had said. A minimum of memory is indispensable, if one is to live really.[27]

Kant saw clearly that the essential human duality is moral autonomy versus physical heteronomy – the freedom of the human will and spirit versus the subjection to the limitations of the human body.[28] The first symptoms of illness make us acutely aware that the body, although simultaneously embodying and expressing our subjective self, is a frail, decaying and frequently dysfunctional object over which we feel ourselves to have no control. With worsening illness, physical heteronomy becomes more and more constraining and, as this happens, the essential limitlessness of moral autonomy becomes more and more important. Doctors need to foster that autonomy and, in some sense, accompany it. Yet too often, we constrain it through a failure of words, a lack of attention or inappropriate or even unwelcome sedation. Pellegrino describes healing as:

> . . . to restore wholeness or, if this is not possible, to assist in striking some new balance between what the body imposes and the self aspires to.[29]

Nothing demonstrates more clearly the lack of connection between healing and cure, and that healing within dying is precisely what we, as both patients and doctors, should be seeking to achieve.

When the weakness and fatigue of dying take someone beyond words, only one side of the conversation is lost. Too often both sides peter out together, but it is important that those around the dying person continue to talk and to express the fullness of their feelings and appreciation for the person who is dying. The ability to hear and understand persists long after the ability to articulate words, and the sharing of memories and the processes of finding meaning and a sense of achievement can continue until the moment of death and often beyond, bringing solace to all concerned. Music can also bring comfort through the evocation of memory and through the sense music conveys of moving beyond time:

> When time is pulse, as music makes it, eternity is in the gaps between.[30]

TOUCH

The practice of medicine involves three different modalities of appropriate touch, all of which are identified and valued by patients: ordinary social touch including the shaking of hands or the touch of consolation or comfort on the arm or shoulder; touching the site of the symptoms to show that the complaint has been understood; and the various levels of the formal clinical examination.[31] Each of these modalities takes place within a context that defines the meaning of the touch. Carl Edvard Rudebeck writes about the way in which exactly the same physical sensation of a hand touching you on the shoulder is interpreted completely differently if it is the touch of a loved one at home and when it is the touch of a stranger in a dark street. The same physical input results in completely different physical outputs – one of contentment, the other of panic.[32] Rudebeck links this to the fact that the lateral geniculate nucleus, the part of the brain which processes vision, draws only 20% of its impulses from the eye and the rest from other parts of the brain that bring the context of memory and history, and allow association and selection to inform the interpretation of what is seen. It seems likely that touch and pain work in the same way. Pain in the context of fear and feeling out of control can be unbearable and overwhelming, whereas pain that is expected and for which there is known to be relief available, if wanted, is much more often bearable.

Like words, touch marks both the separation and the continuity between people,[33] and we need touch to keep communicating when words begin to fail and after they are gone. The touch of someone familiar will always be different from the touch of a stranger.

> However great the kindness and the efficiency, in every hospital death there will be some cruel, squalid detail, something perhaps too small to be told but leaving terribly painful memories behind, arising out of the haste, the crowding, the impersonality of a place where every day people are dying among strangers.[34]

The care of the dying and particularly of those who are no longer able to communicate in words should, as much as possible, be given by those who are known to the patient and preferably by those who are tied with bonds of love. Love makes touch intimate and provides a deeper level of comfort and communication.

> All that the hand says when you touch.[35]

PATIENCE

The absolute unpredictability of the pace of dying is profoundly problematic both for the dying person and for those who try to keep them company.

> It's like he's having his portrait done, his last portrait, no flattering, no prettying, and no one knows how long it will take. Two weeks, three. Nothing to do but sit still and be who you are.[36]

Not knowing whether the process is going to last for months, weeks or hours – not knowing when to say and do things – and then sometimes it's suddenly too late. The uncertainty which is the substrate of living becomes much more acute at the time of dying.

> The principal characteristic of our existence is *suspense*. Nobody – nobody at all – can say how it's going to turn out.[37]

A capacity for patience – the calm abiding of the issue of time[38] – becomes essential. Strength, resilience and hope all fluctuate – waxing and waning unpredictably.

> I was keeping the best for the end, but I don't feel very well, perhaps I'm going, that would surprise me. It is a passing weakness, everyone has experienced that. One weakens, then it passes, one's strength comes back and one resumes.[39]

For those providing care and support, this unpredictability makes it very difficult to judge the timing and intensity of visits and other forms of support, and all the time everyone involved is wondering about tomorrow, about how this process will end.

What shall I die of, in the end?[40]

My mind keeps turning to it . . . you just don't know . . . what it is going to be like. I keep thinking about it . . . you don't know when.

Dermot Donoghue (51 years)[41]

Talking to the relatives and friends of dying people, Michael Young identified the inevitably conflicting feelings that result from this sense of suspense and not knowing:

> Always there was the uncertainty of not knowing how long it would last. Inevitably, there was a conflict in some people's minds between the wish that the dying would never die and the wish that it would be over. Impossible not to think sometimes about the relief that death would bring; impossible not to feel some guilt about thinking it . . .[42]

One answer to this predicament is to foster a heightened sense of involvement and engagement – to explore the depth rather than the duration of time.

Time isn't a question of length. It's a question of depth, isn't it?[43]

Ian McWhinney has emphasised that, unlike other doctors, the general practitioner knows the patient before the disease.[44] General practice provides an opportunity to form relationships with patients while they are relatively well and this provides the solid ground on which to build a coherent response to the illness and disease that comes later. When serious life-threatening disease is diagnosed, the struggle against that disease inevitably becomes the primary focus of the doctor, but when there is no longer any hope of improvement and death is inevitable, it is essential that the focus shifts, once again, back to the unique suffering individual, that the relationship between doctor and patient shifts from the functional 'I–It' to the full intersubjectivity of Martin Buber's 'I–Thou'.[45] 'I–It' relationships treat people as objects to be studied and manipulated for individual or collective ends, and are the foundation of medical science, while 'I–Thou' relationships acknowledge the limitless subjectivity of the other, and in so doing awake and engage the subjectivity of the I. The shift involves real work on the part of the doctor.

It's hard to do a portrait. You must first spend a critical moment in which you quickly – if you're lucky – discard all the commonplaces about the subject of the drawing. More difficult than inventing is giving up accumulated virtues. The things you discovered yesterday are no longer valid. It's impossible to find anything new without first giving something up.[46]

When the disease is winning, it is crucial to see the person again, to rehear and rediscover their individual story, their achievements, hopes and fears – to start again as Frank Auerbach does, scraping the paint away down to the canvas, to make a new portrait of the subject – one that transcends and leaves behind the disease. In doing this, the time of the individual human spirit can be detached from the time of the disease. The time of the disease is deterministic and inexorable, but the time of the person remains their own and dependent on depth and intensity as much as duration.[47]

In reality we are always between two times: that of the body and that of consciousness. Hence the distinction made in all other cultures between body and soul. The soul is first, and above all, the locus of another time.[48]

NOTES AND REFERENCES

1 Hockney D. A wider view. *Modern Painters.* Spring 1998.

2 Sebald WG. *Austerlitz.* London: Penguin Books, 2001, p. 3.

3 Gadamer H-G. *The Enigma of Health.* Palo Alto: Stanford University Press, 1996, p. 98.

4 Tolstoy L. *Anna Karenina* (1875–77). New York: Heritage Press, 1952, p. 567.

5 Taylor W. Monthly Review 1817: LXXXIII; 498. Quoted in: *The Complete Oxford English Dictionary* (2e). Oxford: Oxford University Press, 1989.

6 Berger J. *The Shape of a Pocket.* London: Bloomsbury, 2001, p. 57.

7 Ibid.

8 Berger J. *To the Wedding.* London: Bloomsbury, 1995, p. 87.

9 Berlin I. The decline of Utopian ideas in the West (1978). In: Berlin I. *The Crooked Timber of Humanity.* London: Fontana Press, 1990, p. 38.

10 Daudet A. *In the Land of Pain.* Edited and translated by Julian Barnes. London: Jonathan Cape, 2002, p. 79.

11 Anna Donald, Personal communication, 2003.

12 Eliot TS. Blake. In: *The Sacred Wood: essays on poetry and criticism* (1920). Reprinted in *The Waste Land and Other Writings.* New York: Modern Library, 2002, p. 180.

13 Beckett S. *Malone Dies* (1951). London: Penguin Books, 1962, p. 70.

14 Graves R. The Cool Web. In: *Poems Selected by Himself.* London: Penguin Books, 1966, p. 43. Reprinted by permission of Carcanet Press Ltd.

15 Bakhtin MM. Discourse in the novel (1935). In: *The Dialogic Imagination: four essays.* Austin: University of Texas Press, 1981, p. 259.

16 Borges JL. *This Craft of Verse. The Charles Eliot Norton Lectures 1967–1968.* Cambridge, MA: Harvard University Press, 2000, p. 117.

17 Rudebeck CE. Grasping the existential anatomy: the role of bodily empathy in clinical communication. In: Toombs SK (ed) *Phenomenology and Medicine.* Dordrecht: Kluwer Academic Publishers, 2001.

18 Berger J. Manhattan. In: *The White Bird.* London: The Hogarth Press, 1988, p. 64.

19 Miłosz C. Nobel Lecture, 8 December 1980. http://nobelprize.org/literature/laureates/1980/milosz-lecture-en.html

20 Bakhtin MM. Discourse in the novel (1935). In: *The Dialogic Imagination: four essays*. Austin: University of Texas Press, 1981, p. 300.

21 Borges JL. *This Craft of Verse. The Charles Eliot Norton Lectures 1967–1968*. Cambridge, MA: Harvard University Press, 2000, p. 18.

22 Larkin P. Aubade. In: *Collected Poems*. London: Faber and Faber, 1988, p. 208. Reprinted by permission of Faber and Faber Ltd.

23 Bellow S. What kind of day did you have? In: *Him with his Foot in his Mouth and Other Stories*. London: Penguin Books, 1985, p. 119.

24 Beckett S. *Malone Dies* (1951). London: Penguin Books, 1962, p. 118.

25 Ibid, p. 7.

26 Ibid, p. 94.

27 Ibid, p. 41.

28 Berlin I. The Apotheosis of the Romantic Will. In: *The Crooked Timber of Humanity*. London: Fontana Press, 1990, p. 217.

29 Pellegrino ED. The healing relationship: the architectonics of clinical medicine. In: Shelp EE (ed) *The Clinical Encounter: the moral fabric of the patient–physician relationship*. Dordrecht: Kluwer Academic Publishers, 1983, p. 163.

30 Berger J. *To the Wedding*. London: Bloomsbury, 1995, p. 198.

31 Yee L. *Breaking Barriers: towards culturally competent general practice. A consultation project for the Royal College of General Practitioners' Inner City Task Force*. London: Royal College of General Practitioners, 1997.

32 Rudebeck CE. Grasping the existential anatomy: the role of bodily empathy in clinical communication. In: Toombs SK (ed) *Phenomenology and Medicine*. Dordrecht: Kluwer Academic Publishers, 2001.

33 Berger J. The infinity of desire. *The Guardian*, Thursday July 13, 2000.

34 Orwell G. How the poor die. In: Bamforth I (ed) *The Body in the Library: a literary anthology of modern medicine*. London: Verso, 2003, p. 222.

35 Joyce J. *Ulysses* (1922). London: Penguin Books, 1992, p. 495.

36 Swift G. *Last Orders*. London: Picador, 1996, p. 152.

37 Bellow S. Cousins. In: *Him with his Foot in his Mouth and other Stories*. London: Penguin Books, 1985, p. 237.

38 *Complete Oxford English Dictionary* (2e). Oxford: Oxford University Press, 1989.

39 Beckett S. *Malone Dies* (1951). London: Penguin Books, 1962, p. 97.

40 Ibid, p. 126.

41 Young M and Cullen L. *A Good Death: conversations with East Londoners.* London: Routledge, 1996, p. 91.

42 Young M and Cullen L. *A Good Death: conversations with East Londoners.* London: Routledge, 1996, p. 88.

43 Saunders C, quoted in: Young M and Cullen L. *A Good Death: conversations with East Londoners.* London: Routledge, 1996, p. 120.

44 McWhinney IR. The essence of general practice. In: Lakhani M (ed) *A Celebration of General Practice.* Oxford: Radcliffe Medical Press, 2003.

45 Downie RS and Jodalen H. 'I–Thou' and 'Doctor–Patient': a relationship examined. In: Jodalen H and Vetlesen AJ (eds) *Closeness: an ethics.* Oslo: Scandinavian University Press, 1997, pp. 129–41.

46 Steinberg S with Buzzi A. *Reflections and Shadows.* London: Allen Lane, The Penguin Press, 2001, p. 70.

47 Roy DJ. Waiting for the (un)expected – experiences of time in palliative care. *Journal of Palliative Care.* 1998; 14: 3–4.

48 Berger J. *And our Faces, my Heart, Brief as Photos* (1984) New York: Vintage International, 1991, p. 10.

9 SCIENCE AND POETRY

It is hard to die and it is also difficult to be a doctor: to be confronted every working day with suffering and finitude and a recurring awareness of the limits of science and of one's own skill.[1] When the dying patient meets his or her doctor, both individuals are engaged in one of the most difficult tasks that they will undertake. The doctor has a clear professional responsibility but one which overlaps uncomfortably with the existential tasks of finding love and meaning in the face of suffering and death that are common to all people and for which the doctor has no particular aptitude. It is work that takes place 'in the depths of the body, [where] there is an interface, a shared skin between the physical and metaphysical'.[2] In this situation, it is tough to hold on to the determination to be fully present, not to flinch, not to seek refuge in the detail of bodily symptoms and so avoid confronting fear, anger, grief and loss. Attempting this arduous responsibility, doctors need help and, for me, most help, as I hope I have shown, comes from writers in general and poets in particular.

Poets do the same work of bridging the personal and the universal and they can show doctors, time and again, how it is done:

> It is not an angel
> it is a poet
> he has no wings
> only a right hand
> covered by feathers
> he beats the air with his hand
> flies up three inches
> and immediately falls again
> when he has fallen all the way
> he kicks with his legs
> hangs for a moment
> waving his feathered hand
> oh if he could break from the gravity of clay
> he would dwell in the stars' nest
> he would leap from ray to ray
> he would –
> but at the thought

they would be the earth for him
the stars
fall down in fright
the poet shades his eyes
with his feathered hand
he no longer dreams of flight
but of a fall
that draws like lightning
a profile of infinity.[3]

It is not an angel, it is a doctor. He or she tries and falls short, but both the attempt and the fall are essential parts of the work that he or she must do and it is the fall that accommodates the infinity of the human.

Seamus Heaney writes of:

> . . . a poetry where the co-ordinates of the imagined thing correspond to and allow us to contemplate the complex burden of our own experience.[4]

This captures precisely the gift of the poet – to shed light without simplifying. It is almost exactly the opposite of the gift of science which is to seek understanding through simplification. The complementarity of the two is a thing of wonder, with each having the capacity to enhance the other. Doctors need both science and poetry and never more so than when caring for the dying.

Science has constructed knowledge of the many ways in which the body fails and has allowed humanity to make huge progress in the struggle against death, but when death becomes inevitable and the struggle increasingly futile, science has very little to offer and the resources of poetry become much more important.

I have tried to show how the testimony of poets translates into very practical priorities for the care of people who are dying. Most of these are obvious but need to be constantly restated:

- Whenever possible people should die at home or in another loved and familiar place.
- People should not die alone, and care should be provided by those who are known to the dying person and preferably by those who love them.

- A continuing relationship and conversation between a doctor and a dying patient is essential.
- Communication is mediated by both words and touch.
- Sometimes it is necessary to feel pain, in order to feel alive.
- Hope relates to the future but exists entirely within the present and can be directed towards small sensory pleasures – music, touch, the sight of a loved face, sunshine.
- Reliving and resharing memories allows the completion of a coherent life story.
- Space must be found for acknowledgement of the resolution of a life and the prospect of liberation from a failing body.
- The depth of time is more important than its duration.

As tools for the doctor, these seem simultaneously puny and vast, but if attention is paid to them, it becomes easier not to flinch and thereby to be and to remain present for the patient we will all become.

NOTES AND REFERENCES

1 Barnard D. Love and death: existential dimensions of physicians' difficulties with moral problems. *Journal of Medicine and Philosophy.* 1988; 13: 393–409.

2 Berger J and Trivier M. *My Beautiful.* Douchy-les-Mines: Centre Régional de la Photographie Nord Pas-de-Calais, 2004, p. 31.

3 Herbert Z. Chosen by the stars. In: *Elegy for Departure and other poems.* Hopewell: The Ecco Press, 1999, p. 42. Reprinted by permission of HarperCollins Publishers.

4 Heaney S. *The Redress of Poetry.* London: Faber and Faber Limited, 1995, p. 10.

Twelve Theses on the Economy of the Dead

John Berger

Twelve Theses on the Economy of the Dead

From *Pages of the Wound – poems, drawings, photographs 1956–96*, published by Bloomsbury Circle Press in 1996.

1. The dead surround the living. The living are the core of the dead. In this core are the dimensions of time and space. What surrounds the core is timelessness.

2. Between the core and its surroundings there are exchanges, which are not usually clear. All religions have been concerned with making them clearer. The credibility of religion depends upon the clarity of certain unusual exchanges. The mystifications of religion are the result of trying to systematically produce such exchanges.

3. The rarity of clear exchange is due to the rarity of what can cross intact the frontier between timelessness and time.

4. To see the dead as the individuals they once were tends to obscure their nature. Try to consider the living as we might assume the dead to do: collectively. The collective would accrue not only across space but also throughout time. It would include all those who had ever lived. And so we would also be thinking of the dead. The living reduce the dead to those who have lived; yet the dead already include the living in their own great collective.

5. The dead inhabit a timeless moment of construction continually rebegun. The construction is the state of the universe at any instant.

6. According to their memory of life, the dead know the moment of construction as, also, a moment of collapse. Having lived, the dead can never be inert.

7. If the dead live in a timeless moment, how can they have a memory? They remember no more than being thrown into time, as does everything which existed or exists.

8. The difference between the dead and the unborn is that the dead have this memory. As the number of dead increase, the memory enlarges.

9. The memory of the dead existing in timelessness may be thought of as a form of imagination concerning the possible. This imagination is close to (resides in) God; but I do not know how.

10. In the world of the living there is an equivalent but contrary phenomenon. The living sometimes experience timelessness, as revealed in sleep, ecstasy, instants of extreme danger, orgasm, and perhaps in the experience of dying itself. During these instants the living imagination covers the entire field of experience and overruns the contours of the individual life or death. It touches the waiting imagination of the dead.

11. What is the relation of the dead to what has not yet happened, to the future? All the future *is* the construction in which their 'imagination' is engaged.

12. How do the living live with the dead? Until the dehumanisation of society by capitalism, all the living awaited the experience of the dead. It was their ultimate future. By themselves the living were incomplete. Thus living and dead were inter-dependent. Always. Only a uniquely modern form of egotism has broken this inter-dependence. With disastrous results for the living, we now think of the dead as the *eliminated*.

Connections

Iona Heath

Connections

When I was first asked to consider republishing *The Mystery of General Practice* alongside *Ways of Dying*, I was very uncertain about whether it could make a coherent whole. However, on reflection, it seems that those aspects of general practice that I tried to outline in the *Mystery* are precisely those which are needed when caring for the dying.

When I had the magnificent good fortune to be offered the 1995 Nuffield Trust John Fry Fellowship, I was asked to think about what should not change about general practice and about what we should attempt to defend in times of rapid political and societal change. The result was *The Mystery of General Practice*. Sadly, 12 years on, the roles and potential of general practice seem no better understood by those with political and economic power. Yet, perhaps this is inevitable because the sort of gentle, persistent, undramatic, science-based care at which general practitioners excel is only really valued by the sick, the vulnerable, the frightened and the frail. In relatively prosperous countries, these groups will always tend to be in a relatively easily marginalised minority.

Since 1995, and particularly since the start of the new Labour government in 1997, the pace of organisational change within the National Health Service has accelerated to an extent which is almost certainly counter-productive. The hostility and difficulty of the political context has become, if anything, worse and I did not anticipate the attempts at micro-management mediated by crude financial incentives, the overwhelming culture of inspection and the extent of wasteful duplication of effort that all this has produced. We are no closer to rediscovering a set of values which go beyond the numerical and the financial and the challenge has undoubtedly become more urgent. Nevertheless, despite all, what a fascinating and rewarding undertaking general practice remains.

The extraordinary and encouraging thing is how much of the original text holds true today and it is important to remember how much has not been lost. Everyday, in thousands of consultations across the country, general practitioners work at the interface of illness and disease to resist medicalisation and they continue to acknowledge and witness suffering and endurance. In this context, it is a little disappointing to note that neither of the two key roles that I described are explicitly included within the new curriculum for general practice training.

A more positive change in the intervening years has been the banning of all forms of cigarette advertising and the gradual establishment of smoke-free public places. On the other hand, the state of care for the frail elderly has fulfilled one of my more gloomy prognostications and this was underlined by the failure of the government to implement the recommendations of the Royal Commission on Long Term Care in England. However, the implementation in Scotland was immensely encouraging and has underlined the more robust defence of the solidarity which underpins the National Health Service in Scotland, Wales and Northern Ireland. As these differences become more pronounced, even those living in England may eventually benefit through political pressure based on comparison.

The most significant loss that general practice has sustained is one that I anticipated, but only vaguely. I thought that, under Thatcher, something precious had already been lost but that 'there may be much more to lose'. In 2007, the vast majority of UK general practitioners have given up their responsibility for the care of their patients 24 hours a day and seven days a week and are now contracted to care for their patients from 8 in the morning to 6.30 at night and for only five days a week. Most patients are at a loss to understand why this has been allowed to happen. While there is no doubt that a majority of general practitioners did not want to continue with their obligation to provide 24-hour care, many would have retained responsibility if they had not been financially penalised for doing so. To my mind, there is no doubt that general practice has been damaged by this diminution of responsibility and, perhaps most importantly, it is impossible to provide adequate care for the dying and those around them if one can only be contacted for 10 and a half hours a day, five days a week. Many of my colleagues have discovered that the only feasible way of providing adequate care under current arrangements is to give families our personal mobile phone numbers. Yet, if the care available is not good enough for the dying it is almost certainly not good enough for anyone who is seriously ill and in danger of being overwhelmed by fear. This is the link between the two parts of this book – the challenge of caring for the dying provides the crucial test of general practice and general practitioners.

Iona Heath
September 2007

The Mystery of
General Practice

Iona Heath

The Mystery of General Practice

THE JOHN FRY TRUST FELLOWSHIP

When he retired in 1991, after 45 years as a general practitioner, Dr John Fry established a Trust, the main aim of which was to further the development of primary health care.

Through this Trust a Fellowship was established to be awarded annually to a distinguished individual from any discipline. Each holder of the Fellowship would be invited to prepare a monograph which it was hoped would contribute significantly to the progress of primary care. The monograph would be introduced by a public lecture to be delivered at a recognised teaching centre in the United Kingdom.

ACKNOWLEDGEMENTS

I owe an enormous debt to the many patients, friends and colleagues who have taught me about general practice over the years. In the preparation of this monograph, I am grateful to Godfrey Fowler for his belief in me, to Michael Ashley-Miller for his consistent support and encouragement, and to David Morrell and Carl Edvard Rudebeck for their reassurance. In particular, I wish to thank Stephen Amiel and Duncan Keeley for their painstaking criticisms of earlier drafts. Typically, I have resisted some of their advice and the remaining faults are my own. Most of all, I thank David Heath for tirelessly reading and commenting on every draft, for his belief that I had something to say and for doing much more than his share of the ironing.

Contents

1 INTRODUCTION

Sadly, I did not have the opportunity to know John Fry well, but I did have the privilege to serve with him on the Council of the Royal College of General Practitioners during the last year of his thirty-year tenure. John Fry made a unique contribution to general practice research through the careful recording of his daily work in Beckenham. I have no credentials in research, but I do aspire to share with John Fry a love of ordinary general practice and a firm belief in its power to improve the health of individuals and populations.[1]

My title came originally from my delight in discovering that a mystery was an early collective noun for doctors. An archaic meaning of a 'mystery' was 'a trade, profession or calling', and, as such, a mystery was used to describe a faculty of our precursors, the barber-surgeons, in the late middle ages.

Within its more usual meaning,[2] mystery is the subject of this monograph. The mysterious secrets of the trade or art of general practice seem to be poorly understood outside our discipline and, in the face of the current avalanche of change, there is an increasingly urgent need for us to explain ourselves. Carl Edvard Rudebeck, writing about the struggle to establish and develop general practice in Sweden,[3] argues:

> General practice was pushed into defining itself at its own margins, leaving its very centre, its specific priorities, unfathomed by both critics and spokesmen.

Here in the UK we have the same problem. The pace of change has been rapid and seems to be accelerating. We are continually having to adapt our practice and our attitudes, and in so doing we tend to lose sight of those parts of our work which should not change because they deal with enduring aspects of the human experience of illness and disease.[4] Unless we are able to make our specific contribution explicit we will not be valued and we may be lost.

We might ask why the key transactions of general practice are mysterious. I suspect that it is because they have developed out of an inarticulate mix of intuition and experience, and that we only slowly begin to understand them ourselves when we embark in practice as young doctors. We research, teach and learn about the dynamics of the consultation but, somehow, often continue to assume, rather than explain, the nature of the fundamental transactions.

This monograph begins with some of the components of the current malaise in general practice, and after a brief discussion of the nature of medicine, goes on to attempt to lay open the secrets, mystery and particular contribution of general practice. In so doing, I hope to demonstrate the crucial value of general practice, to define the prerequisites for, and the threats to, its survival and to argue the case for its active perpetuation through education and research.

NOTES AND REFERENCES

1 Fry J and Horder J. *Primary Health Care in an International Context.* London: Nuffield Provincial Hospitals Trust, 1994.

2 Definitions of mystery given in the Oxford English Dictionary include:
'A hidden or secret thing; a matter unexplained or inexplicable.' 'The behaviour or attitude of mind of one who makes a secret of things usually for the purpose of exercising undue power or influence.' 'An action or practice about which there is or is supposed to be a secret or highly technical operation in a trade or art.'

3 Rudebeck CE. General practice and the dialogue of clinical practice: on symptoms, symptom presentations and bodily empathy. *Scand J Prim Health Care.* 1992; Suppl 1.

4 Willis J. *The Paradox of Progress.* Oxford: Radcliffe Medical Press, 1995.

2 THE CURRENT CRISIS

It is now five years since the government imposed changes on the National Health Service, introducing almost simultaneously the purchaser-provider split and the New Contract for General Practice. These changes have precipitated a crisis in the morale of general practitioners and a fall in the number of applicants to join general practice training schemes. More recently, the Department of Health has called for the development of a primary care-led NHS.[1] General practitioners are being asked to extend their role in many different directions and there is a feeling that politicians and health service planners are seeking to place general practice at the centre of the NHS without properly understanding the essential transactions of its displine.[2] Throughout the profession, there has been a perceived need to rediscover core values[3] and this has been particularly marked in general practice.[4] This need must derive from a sense of threat, a feeling that in adapting to the avalanche of change we are in danger of losing something precious, something that once lost will be difficult, if not impossible, to regain. That something seems to be concerned with the intimate interaction between the individual patient and the generalist doctor and I will discuss this in detail later. First it is necessary to address those developments which are both undermining and distracting attention from the essential nature of general practice.

MARKET VALUES AND THE DESTRUCTION OF VOCATION

By introducing market values into the transaction of health care and turning patients into consumers, while at the same time putting strict limits on the resources available, the Government has trapped health workers in the credibility gap between rhetoric and reality. Charters offer a superficial vision of quality which has everything to do with being a consumer but very little to do with the needs priorities and responsibilities of being a patient. Most patients understand John Howle's[5] definition:

> Effectiveness is the ability to justify extra time spent on one patient in terms of the cost imposed on all succeeding patients.

Patients recognise that moments of crisis, such as collapse, bereavement or the communication of a serious diagnosis, require extra time and most are prepared to meet the cost in the belief that they will benefit at their own moment of crisis. This is not the logic of the consumer or the market.[6] Markets thrive on individual gratification, which is devoid of a social context. They are linked to a form of politics which seeks to minimise not only taxation but also the obligation to invest in social justice.

For us as health workers, every component of health care appears now to have its price – we are exhorted to consider the financial implications of our every action. Not surprisingly this has led us in our turn to consider the financial value attributed to our work and this has resulted in an attrition of vocation. The 'Out of Hours' story tells much of this. Patients are turned into consumers and given rising expectations of what they have a right to expect, doctors are turned into purveyors of a commodity rather than members of a vocational profession providing a public service.[7] Patients begin to ask for medical attention at night for worries which could wait until the following day. Doctors begin to look at precisely what they are paid for offering a 24-hour service 365 days of the year and they find that it is very little for the discomfort of having to get out of a warm bed after a long day's work and with the prospect of another one only a few hours away.

By failing to value the notion of professional vocation, our society is allowing it to wither away. This is something precious which seems already lost; there may be much more to lose. Thatcherism's most dangerous legacy may prove to be this erosion of professional and vocational motivation and its replacement by the single-minded pursuit of financial and material reward. Such self-seeking has become the acceptable norm and the great challenge for the future is to rediscover a sense of vocation and of society.

THE CONFLICT BETWEEN ADVOCACY AND DISTRIBUTIVE JUSTICE

General practitioners are increasingly aware of the conflict between their role as the individual patient's advocate on the one hand, and, on the other, their increasing role in decisions about the distribution of scarce resources within a population. The trust of the patient depends on their belief that their general practitioner understands and empathises with the needs they express and this impels and empowers the general practitioner to act as the patient's advocate. This advocacy role inevitably conflicts with involvement in decisions about the distribution of limited resources. It is not possible to strive simultaneously for the individual and the collective good. The two are based on quite distinct ethical principles and there will always be problems when collective principles are applied to the care of individuals.[8] The problem is acknowledged by the Chief Medical Officer:[9]

> It may be necessary to separate decision making at the bedside from resource allocation at a higher level.

And yet the pressure on general practitioners to become fundholders is intense. The conflict of interest must be understood for the profound dilemma that it is and not dismissed as a shirking of responsibility by those general practitioners who, in a time of shrinking resources, increasing need and ideologically inflated demand, refuse to engage in what is effectively bedside rationing.

THE SPECIOUS SEPARATION OF HEALTH CARE AND SOCIAL CARE

The current Community Care arrangements are founded on the conviction that it is possible to distinguish between health and social care, but in reality the demarcation is illusory. Anyone who is so frail that they are unable to provide their own personal care has self-evident health needs. For general practitioners (and for patients) health and social care form a continuum and the debate about the distribution of responsibility and resources across the fictitious boundary is fundamentally flawed. Unfortunately the present state of the law decrees that health care should be provided free at the point of delivery, whereas social care can be charged to the patient or their family. When resources are insufficient this leads to pressure to define needs as social and to pass the costs of care on to the patient.

The difficulties for the patient concern the well-recognised poverty trap and the emerging 'disability trap'. Charges for social care services are applied to anyone in possession of more than a very small capital sum, and this includes property even if it is still occupied by other members of the family. Those without capital and receiving Income Support have the full cost of their care provided but others, particularly those just above the threshold, face considerable difficulties. Families can find themselves faced with a sequence of losses, a parent's health followed by the family home.

The disability trap is even more insidious. Faced with inadequate resources, local authorities are having to choose between providing some level of input to large numbers of frail and dependent people or a more intensive and expensive service to only the most dependent. Most feel obliged to choose the latter, with the result that people are denied help until they have fallen below a threshold set at a standard of care that many find quite unacceptable. Once services are provided, they are usually of a high standard but the phase of deterioration to the qualifying level is distressing, humiliating and destructive of families.[10]

For doctors, and other members of the primary care team, efforts to deliver a high standard of health care in a context of inadequate social care often prove futile. The process is akin to trying to fill a bucket without a bottom and the net effect is to sap the morale of both patients and health workers.

HEALTH PROMOTION INSTEAD OF HEALTH PROTECTION

The tidal wave of health promotion rhetoric seems, from position in inner-city general practice, to be an elaborate mechanism for blaming the victims.[11] In 1812, the poet Shelley[12] described the same injustice:

> The rich grind the poor into abjectness and then complain that they are abject.

Cigarette smoking is the key example. I believe that all my patients are now fully informed of the dangers of smoking. Sadly many continue to smoke because they lead lives which are so materially and emotionally constrained that cigarette smoking is one of pitifully few sources of pleasure and relief. All the evidence tells us that banning cigarette advertising would do more to reduce the levels of cigarette smoking in this country than any other measure and yet it is not done, for purely fiscal reasons. Health differentials based on social class are blamed on lifestyle choices, the victims are blamed, and the responsibility for reducing cigarette smoking is passed to the general practitioner who must raise the subject, to the point of becoming very tedious, on every possible occasion.[13] Shah Ebrahlm[14] draws the distinction between health promotion, which is a responsibility of health workers, and health protection, which is a responsibility of government. The government has pursued the rhetoric of health promotion to disguise its failure in the arena of health protection. Patients are deprived twice over; first by the absence of adequate health protection measures and then by the erosion of time within the consultation by the ever-increasing health promotion agenda.[15]

All general practitioners, to a greater or lesser extent, are disturbed by these developments. We struggle with the ethical dilemmas they impose and we complain. They are eroding of the essential nature of general practice. Further, they distract us from the more fundamental questions which are at the heart of our unease. These questions are about the nature of medicine and our particular role as generalists within the large endeavour of the discipline of medicine.

NOTES AND REFERENCES

1 NHS Executive. *Developing NHS Purchasing and GP Fundholding*. Leeds: NHS Executive, 1994.

2 Metcalfe D. Care in the capital: what needs to be done. *British Medical Journal*. 1992; **305**: 1141–4.

3 BMA Secretariat. *Core Values for the Medical Profession in the 21st Century*. London: BMA, 1995.

4 Joint Working Party of the Welsh Council of the Royal College of General Practitioners and the Welsh General Medical Services Committee. Patient care and the general practitioner. *British Medical Journal*. 1994; **309**: 1144–7.

5 Howie J. Personal communication, 1990.

6 Dunstan GR. *Ideology, Ethics and Practice*. London: RCGP, 1994.

7 McWhinney I. *A Textbook of Family Medicine*. Oxford: Oxford University Press, 1989.
'Human variability is such that for a seriously ill person, the physician cannot be a replaceable part. If we insist on treating ourselves as such, we should not be surprised if society treats us as laborers rather than as professionals. We should also not be surprised if it does something to us as people. As we withdraw from our patients we will be poorer for it. Our professional lives will be less satisfying, and we will lose much of the depth of experience that medicine will give us.'

8 Veatch RM. Justice in health care: the contribution of Edmund Pellegrino. *J Med Phil*. 1990; **15**: 269–87.

9 Calman K. The profession of medicine. *British Medical Journal*. 1994; **309**: 1140–3.

10 Ellis K. *Squaring the Circle: user and carer participation in needs assessment*. York: Joseph Rowntree Foundation, 1993.

11 Marantz PR. Blaming the victim: the negative consequence of preventive medicine. *Am J Pub Health*. 1990; **80**(10): 1186–7.

12 Quoted in: Holmes R. *Shelley: the pursuit*. London: Weidenfeld & Nicolson, 1974.

13 Stott NCH, Kinnersley P and Rollnick S. The limits to health promotion. *British Medical Journal*. 1994; 309: 971–2.

14 Ebrahim S. *Public health implications of ageing*. Milroy Lecture. London: Royal College of Physicians, 1994.

15 Sullivan F. Intruders in the consultation. *Fam Pract*. 1995; 12: 66–9.

3 NATURE OF MEDICINE

The story of medicine is one of striving to make sense of the human experience of illness. Patients who perceive themselves to be ill have always asked questions of the doctor:[1] 'Am I indeed ill?' 'Can I be cured?' 'Can my suffering be relieved?' 'Why has this happened to me?' 'What will happen to me now?' 'Will I die?' The enormous advances of scientific medicine over the last century have meant affirmative answers to the second question – 'Can I be cured?' – in more and more cases with much relief of suffering and prevention of premature death. However, this has been at the cost of avoiding the other questions and the human need is for all the questions to be answered. Medicine is diminished by too narrow a definition of the discipline, in terms both of the nature of illness and disease, and of their causes.

THE NATURE OF ILLNESS AND DISEASE

Illness begins as a subjective sense of bodily unease, an experience of the functioning of the body as being not quite right.[2] It is often very intangible and the sense of unease arises not just from what we have come to recognise as disease but also from other forms of distress including tiredness and unhappiness, misery and grief. With the success of scientific medicine has come an emphasis on disease which has tended to invalidate the individual's experience of illness. Distress and unease which do not fit into a pattern of disease that science has taught us to recognise are belittled and ignored.

THE CAUSES OF ILLNESS AND DISEASE

The wider causes of illness and ultimately of disease are also ignored in too narrow a definition of disease. Many doctors and politicians have been reluctant to recognise the power and extent of the socio-economic determinants of ill-health; the ways in which society functions to make its own members unwell through the stresses of poverty, poor housing, unemployment, pollution and lack of opportunity for worthwhile achievement. Ordinary people seem always to have known these things – ask them what is important to their health and they will mention housing, safety and opportunity for their children, adequate income and opportunities for work. Yet, *The Health of the*

Nation[3] minimised the impact of poverty[4] and completely failed to mention the influence of unemployment on health.[5]

THE MYTH OF CURE

The welcome success of scientific medicine carries other dangers. The chief of these is the implication, the false promise, that science offers a cure for every ill and the indefinite postponement of death.[6] Death, which is inevitable, and often unpredictable, arbitrary and unjust, is seen more and more as a simple failure of medicine and doctors. Medicine cannot promise immortality and yet we, in Western society, begin to convince ourselves that it might. Neither does it promise the relief of all bodily discomfort and pain, and yet we become less and less tolerant of these and more convinced that we have a right to perfect health. Scientists and doctors carry a great responsibility for perpetuating these dangerous illusions,[7] which serve to further damage, demoralise, stigmatise and disappoint victims of the many chronic diseases which can be treated but not cured and whose sufferers must often pay a high price in terms of discomfort, restrictions and inconvenience.[8]

The emphasis on lifestyle risk factors for disease creates a climate of victim-blaming which adds a sense of guilt[9] to the distress and terror suffered by those arbitrarily afflicted by serious disease. Arthur Kleinmanl[10] reminds us that:

> Cancer is an unsettling reminder of the obdurate grain of unpredictability and uncertainty and injustice – value questions, all – in the human condition.

Similarly intractable is the kind of chronic illness which seems to arise from profound and insoluble unhappiness, and manifests itself in, for example, continuous fatigue, aching muscles, insomnia, palpitations and frustration. Scientific medicine has offered so little here and its successes distract attention away from what might be achieved by a fairer, more equitable society within which the rewards of human life and endeavour would be more evenly shared.

THE SEARCH FOR MEANING

Where we cannot cure we must be available to help the patient to make some kind of sense of their suffering. In such circumstances, the need for answers to the last four questions becomes overwhelming: 'Can my suffering be relieved?' 'Why has this happened to me?' 'What will happen to me now?' 'Will I die?'

The general practitioner, often seeing patients through 20 or 30 years of illness and disease, both major and minor, as well as a series of significant life events, is in a unique position to help the patient make some kind of sense of what is happening to them. The key skill here is to listen and in so doing to allow the patient to find their own pattern and explanation. The doctor witnesses the suffering, the struggle and the fortitude of the patient and the relationship is one of solidarity. The patient is allowed and enabled to tell the story of their illness to the doctor during a succession of consultations which may extend over many years.[11] During this process the patient's burden is shared and their experience is validated by being recounted to an external witness provided by society, in the person of the doctor.[12]

Peter Toon[13] states:

> The consultation is the patient's forum for coming to understand her illness; not merely a rational understanding, but an understanding which involves the emotions and which contributes to the growth of the individual.

I have argued that the second illness question 'Can I be cured?' may be answered by scientific medicine. The first 'Am I indeed ill?' is the forum of co-operative endeavour between patient and general practitioner and provides the latter with a key role. The remaining four – 'Can my suffering be relieved?', 'Why has this happened to me?', 'What will happen to me now?', 'Will I die?' – are answered partly by science and partly within the search for meaning. Accompanying the patient in this search provides the doctor with another key role.

NOTES AND REFERENCES

1 Helman CG. Disease versus illness in general practice. *J Roy Coll Gen Pract.* 1981; 31: 548–52. My questions are different but my debt clear.

2 Rudebeck CE. General practice and the dialogue of clinical practice: on symptoms, symptom presentations and bodily empathy. *Scand J Prim Health Care.* 1992; Suppl 1.

3 Department of Health. *The Health of the Nation: a strategy for health in England.* London: HMSO, 1992.

4 Wilkinson RG. Income distribution and life expectancy. *British Medical Journal.* 1992; **304**: 165–8.

5 Beale N and Nethercott S. The nature of unemployment morbidity. *J Roy Coll Gen Pract.* 1988; **38**: 197–202.

6 McCormick J. Fifty years of progress. *J Roy Coll Gen Pract.* 1975; **25**: 9–19.

7 Tallis R. Medical advances and the future of old age. In: Marinker M (ed) *Controversies in Health Care Policies: challenges to practice.* London: BMJ Publishing Group, 1994.

8 Heaney S. *The Cure at Troy.* Derry: Field Day Theatre Company, 1990.

9 Bennett MI and Bennett MB. The uses of hopelessness. *Am J Psychiatry.* 1984; **141**: 559–62.

10 Kleinman A. *The Illness Narratives: suffering, healing and the human condition.* New York: Basic Books, 1988.

11 Williams GH and Wood PN. Common-sense beliefs about illness: a mediating role for the doctor. *Lancet.* 1986; **2**: 1435–7.

12 Berger J and Mohr J. *A Fortunate Man: the story of a country doctor.* Harmondsworth: Allen Lane, The Penguin Press, 1967.

13 Toon P. *What is good general practice?* Occasional Paper 65. Exeter: RCGP, 1994.

4 THE KEY ROLES OF GENERAL PRACTICE

In 1974, the Leeuwenhorst Working Party of European general practitioners devised the following familiar description of general practice:

> The general practitioner is a licensed medical graduate who gives care to individuals, irrespective of age, sex and illness. He will attend his patients in his consulting room and in their homes and sometimes in a clinic or a hospital. His aim is to make early diagnoses. He will include and integrate physical, psychological, and social factors in his considerations about health and illness. He will make an initial decision about every problem which is presented to him as a doctor. He will undertake the continuing management of his patients with chronic, recurrent or terminal illnesses. Prolonged contact means that he can use repeated opportunities to gather information at a pace appropriate to each patient and build up a relationship of trust which he can use professionally. He will practice in co-operation with other colleagues, medical and non-medical. He will know how and when to intervene through treatment, prevention and education to promote the health of his patients and their families. He will recognize that he also has a professional responsibility to the community.

This definition is trapped in its time by its irritating use of an exclusive pronoun and by its lack of reference to cultural factors but it remains a useful definition to which we continue to aspire. Taken together with the original, absurdly idealistic, 1946 WHO definition of health as:

> a state of complete physical, mental and social wellbeing,[1] and not merely the absence of disease or infirmity

it underpins the essential generalism of general practitioner care. All aspects of human existence are legitimate concerns of the general practitioner provided that they are presented as a problem by the patient. This means that the general practitioner is obliged to deal with the complexity of each individual patient and should never be content to respond to a patient by saying, 'That's not my business or my problem.'[2] Each person and each context is unique and this is the joy and the challenge of general practitioner care.

Making full use of this breadth, the key roles of the general practitioner are firstly to serve as interpreter and guardian at the interface between illness and disease; and secondly to serve as a witness to the patient's experience of illness and disease.

The pivotal position of British general practice arose out of a nineteenth century trade demarcation dispute between physicians and surgeons on the one hand and apothecaries on the other.[3] The physicians and surgeons gained absolute control of the great hospitals being built in every major city by letting the apothecaries have the patients. This was done by instituting the referral process by which the hospital specialists agreed only to see patients who were referred to them by the generalist apothecaries. This fortuitous outcome has been one of the great successes of the British health care system and the foundation of its widely recognised cost-effectiveness. Systems which have developed without a referral process between generalist and specialist have now recognised the need to create one. Specialist care is vastly more expensive than generalist care and by controlling access via a generalist who is able to treat 90% of all illness episodes presented costs can be much more effectively contained.[4]

The cost effectiveness of this boundary between generalist and specialist is recognised and valued but the importance of the interface between illness and disease is much less understood. This is the point at which the vast, undifferentiated mass of human distress and suffering meets the theoretical structures of scientific medicine and the social sciences which have been developed to enable humanity, to a still very limited extent, to understand and control the experience of illness. The illness is the patient's perception of something being wrong, the sense of unease in the functioning of the body or mind; the disease is a defined entity which offers the benefits and risks of scientific medicine. Illness is what the patient has on their way to see the doctor and a disease is what they have on the way home. The former is subjective, the latter objective. Most disease involves illness, but by no means all illness involves disease. Both the disease and the illness can be more or less serious. The task of the general practitioner is to make these distinctions and to diagnose disease, to refer serious treatable disease to specialist colleagues, to treat less serious disease and to acknowledge and witness the suffering brought by illness.

Interpretation at the interface between illness and disease offers the answer to the first question: 'Am I ill?', and the implicit supplementary questions:

'And might I be so ill that I might die?', 'Or am I just distressed?' The way the construction of the words overlaps is fascinating – dis-ease, un-ease, dis-stress, stress. The overenthusiastic interpretation of illness as disease, borne of inexperience or fear of litigation, leaves patients open to the dangers but not the benefits of scientific medicine. Arthur Kleinman[5] writes:

> The physician's training also encourages the dangerous fallacy of over-literal interpretation of accounts best understood metaphorically.

The demise of religious and philosophical explanations for the arbitrariness of human suffering has left the modern world with limited means of understanding and coping. Illness is one of the few valid outlets for human distress. But if that illness is wrongly interpreted as disease all kinds of damage can be done. Thus the first role includes elements of both interpreter and guardian.[6] The general practitioner as interpreter engages the patient in the necessary dialogue. The general practitioner as guardian safeguards the patient from the too ready interpretation of illness as disease. This guardian role is a parallel and prerequisite to the more widely acknowledged role as gatekeeper between primary and secondary care.

Carl Edvard Rudebeck,[7] has developed this argument further. He defines the core skill of general practice as bodily empathy. This is the ability to identify imaginatively with the patient's subjective experience of illness to provide genuine recognition and validation of that experience. Only if the patient can believe that their experience is understood at a fundamental level by the doctor will that patient be able to trust in the doctor's interpretation of their illness. He distinguishes the subjective experience of 'body-as-self' from the objective experience of 'body-as-nature'. As doctors, we combine the subjective experience of our own bodies and minds, with the objective theoretical understanding of the science of their working. By straddling this divide within his or her own body, the generalist doctor is qualified to interpret the interface between illness and disease.[8]

The depth of understanding involved in this interpretation begins the process of witnessing, in which the doctor works with the patient to make sense of the patient's experience of both illness and disease in the context of the rest of their lives. This is what Peter Toon has called the hermeneutic role,[9] and Marshall Marinker, the biographic role. All of us need our experience and, most of all, our sufferings to be acknowledged and given value; we need to tell our stories and have them heard. As doctors we enjoy the enormous privilege of witnessing the experience not only of our own lives but parts of those of all our patients.

The last of the illness questions is 'Will I die?' and an essential test of the doctor is to what extent we are prepared to accompany the patient in their search for an answer. Scientific medicine has allowed doctors to escape from their traditional role as 'the familiar of death', but to do so is to betray the role of witness. John Berger recognises this:

> The doctor is the familiar of death. When we call for a doctor, we are asking him to cure us and to relieve our suffering, but, if he cannot cure us, we are also asking him to witness our dying. The value of the witness is that he has seen so many others die . . . He is the living intermediary between us and the multitudinous dead. He belongs to us and he has belonged to them. And the hard but real comfort which they offer through him is still that of fraternity.

Petr Skrabanek has argued that we have lost touch with the art of dying[10] coincident with beginning to value longevity more than the intensity of the experience of living. He quotes John Stuart Mill's 'Utility of Religion':

> It is not, naturally and generally, the happy who are most anxious either for prolongation of the present life or for a life hereafter; it is those who have never been happy.

By refamiliarising ourselves with death, we can undo some of the mischievous damage that science has done with its illusory promise of immortality. We have an obligation to debate with our patients and society the limitations as well as the possibilities of medicine.[11]

THE CONSULTATION

The consultation is the foundation of general practice:

> the occasion when in the intimacy of the consulting room, or the sick room, a person who is ill or believes himself to be ill, seeks the advice of a doctor whom he trusts.[12]

This occasion provides the opportunity for the patient's story to be heard and for their experience to be acknowledged. If this is done well the enormous benefits of scientific medicine can be made available and the dangers minimised. Julian Tudor Hart[13] moves beyond the rather paternalistic notion of advice and describes the consultation as a unit of production enacted between two co-producers of health – the patient and the doctor – in a meeting of experts. He writes:

> Unless consultations are understood as the points of production of critically important decisions which determine all other consumptions, the cost-effectiveness of the entire NHS will fall in terms of net health gain, even if it improves in terms of reduced waiting times or raised outputs of technical procedures. The quality of consultations must in large part depend on freedom from time pressures, without perverse incentives to save time by ill-considered somatisation, prescription or referral, and with protected time in which to develop patients' capacities as producers rather than consumers.

The consultation provides the setting for the key transactions of general practice. I have argued that the key roles are to serve as an interpreter and guardian at the interface between illness and disease, and to serve as a witness to the illness experience. These roles discharge a crucial social function to the extent that in circumstances when they are unfilled, the individual and collective experience of illness and disease is harsher and more lonely, and humanity is the meaner.[14] These key roles of general practice require a particular combination of skills and circumstances, the continued availability of which is necessary to the survival of the discipline.

NOTES AND REFERENCES

1 With justification, this has been mocked by Skrabanek as 'The sort of feeling ordinary people may achieve fleetingly during orgasm, or when high on drugs.' Skrabanek P. *The Death of Humane Medicine and the Rise of Coercive Healthism*. London: Social Affairs Unit, London, 1994.

2 McWhinney IR. *A Textbook of Family Medicine*. New York: Oxford University Press, 1989.
'Family medicine does not separate disease from person or person from environment.'

3 Marinker M. *The end of general practice*. Bayliss Lecture. London: Royal College of Physicians, 1994.

4 Fry J and Horder J. *Primary Health Care in an International Context*. London: Nuffield Provincial Hospitals Trust, 1994.

5 Kleinman A. *The Illness Narratives: suffering, healing and the human condition*. New York: Basic Books, 1988.

6 Heath I. The future of general practice. In: Lock S (ed) *Eighty-five Not Out: essays to honour Sir George Godber*. London: King Edward's Hospital Fund for London, 1993.

7 Rudebeck CE. General practice and the dialogue of clinical practice: symptoms, symptom presentations and bodily empathy. *Scand J Prim Health Care*. 1992; Suppl 1.

8 Berger J and Mohr J. *A Fortunate Man: the story of a country doctor*. Harmondsworth: Allen Lane, The Penguin Press, 1967.
'It is the doctor's acceptance of what the patient tells him and the accuracy of his appreciation as he suggests how different parts of his life may fit together; it is this which then persuades the patient that he and the doctor and other men are comparable because whatever he says of himself or his fears or his fantasies seems to be at least as familiar to the doctor as to him. He is no longer an exception. He can be recognised. And this is the prerequisite for cure or adaptation.'

9 Toon P. *What is good general practice?* Occasional Paper 65. Exeter: RCGP, 1994.

10 Ignatieff M. *The Needs of Strangers.* London: Chatto & Windus, 1984.
'Most other cultures, including many primitive ones whom we have subjugated to our reason and our technology, enfold their members dying as in an art of living. But we have left these awesome tasks of culture to private choice.'

11 Armstrong EM. We must not let science blind us. *BMA News Review.* 1995; March 8.

12 Spence J. *The Purpose and Practice of Medicine.* Oxford: Oxford University Press, 1960.

13 Hart JT. *Feasible Socialism: the National Health Service, past, present and future.* London: Socialist Health Association, 1994.

14 Thomasma DC. Establishing the moral basis of medicine: Edmund D Pellegrino's philosophy of medicine. *J Med Phil.* 1990; **15**: 245–67.

5 WHAT IS NEEDED

The consultation brings together the human experience of suffering and the paradigms of scientific medicine, with the general practitioner acting as an interpreter at the boundary between illness and disease, and a witness to suffering. In order to fulfill these roles effectively, general practitioners must work from a firm foundation of clinical competence. Without this, we betray our patients' trust and become dangerous. Beyond it we need generalism, continuity, empathy, words, partisanship, time and trust.

We must be generalists acknowledging all forms of distress as legitimate, and we need to be able to provide continuity of care over time. We must have the time and the skill to listen and to hear, to the extent of being able to empathise, so the patient feels understood and is able to trust. We need to be able to find words which demonstrate our understanding. We must become partisans, consistently choosing to side with our patients.

As general practitioners, we need the ability to identify imaginatively with a wide range of individuals. To achieve this we need to avail ourselves of as wide an experience of humanity as possible[1] and borrow skills from other disciplines.[2] We must make available the benefits of scientific medicine but mitigate its dangers through an understanding of anthropology, biography, poetry, myth, philosophy and politics. The skills of anthropology and biography help us with empathy and the use of continuity, and an awareness of poetry and myth can help us find the words to communicate our understanding to the patient. A grasp of philosophy and politics can show us how to be effective partisans on behalf of our patients.

SHARED HISTORY, BIOGRAPHY AND ANTHROPOLOGY

Richard Holmes, the biographer of Shelley and Coleridge, has described the need for everyone to tell their story[3] and to have it valued.

> I learned how much everyone needs to talk about their own past, the forces and experiences that shaped them . . . and how rarely this constant need is satisfied in the competitive, pressurised world, except in moments of emotional crisis.

and:

. . . the lives of great artists and poets and writers are not, after all, so extraordinary by comparison with everyone else. Once known in any detail and any scope, every life is something extraordinary, full of particular drama and tension and surprise, often containing unimagined degrees of suffering or heroism, and invariably touching extreme moments of triumph and despair, though frequently unexpressed. The difference lies in the extent to which one is eventually recorded, and the other is eventually forgotten.

This resonates so clearly with the experience of general practice. To a greater or lesser degree, we all serve as the biographers of our patients,[4] of that portion of their lives which they choose to share with us.

I have been in practice in Kentish Town in north London since 1975 and in that time I have moved, alongside some of my patients, from my 20s to my 40s. We have been replaced by those I first knew as babies. Other patients have moved from their 40s to their 60s or from their 60s to their 80s. These are progressions which involve many changes and much experience, and over the years these patients have shared their histories with me. In a professional span of 35 years, a general practitioner can expect to see patients through almost half a lifetime and this continuity is a powerful tool.[5] It contrasts sharply with the contemporary world of short-term contracts and episodic care. Within this new world, managers, who increasingly define our working conditions, are almost all on short-term contracts and setting themselves increasingly short-term objectives. Health workers are judged in terms of their caseload throughput and by the number of completed episodes of care they deliver. General practitioners are now almost unique in being spared the pressure to discharge patients from a caseload. We alone retain the benefit of continuity and remain free to work within the extended timescale of chronic illness.

General practitioners are privileged to have a part in their patients' experience of family changes, retirement from work, move of home, illness, death and loss. This shared experience forms a bond of trust and respect which is mutual and earned over time. This trust allows the doctor and the patient to work together in their task of making sense of illness experience.[6] It also provides the context for the diagnosis of disease. It is only by following the patient through the whole of their illness experience, both the mundane and the extraordinary, that we can hope to recognise the serious diagnosis 'lurking in the shadow cast by . . . interminable complaining'.[7] It is the ability to recognise that, on this occasion, the complaint is qualitatively different.

WORDS, POETRY AND MYTH

The meanings of illness, the threat, the fear, the suffering and the endurance can only be interpreted, ordered and contained if both doctors and patients can find and agree on the right words. Michael Ignatieff[8] writes:

> We need words to keep us human . . . Our needs are made of words: they come to us in speech, and they die for lack of expression. Without a public language to help us find our own words, our needs will dry up in silence. It is words only, the common meanings they bear, which give me the right to speak in the name of the strangers at my door. Without a language adequate to this moment we risk losing ourselves in resignation towards the portion of life which has been allotted to us. Without the light of language, we risk becoming strangers to our better selves.

By expression in words the communication between doctor and patient becomes explicit. Only if the doctor can find words which the patient recognises as describing his or her own experience, can the patient be certain that he or she has been understood.

There are strong parallels with poetry and we have much to learn from poets, with whom we share:

> . . . the desire to witness exactly.[9]

Seamus Heaney describes poetry as:

> . . . a point of entry into the buried life of the feelings or as a point of exit for it. Words themselves are doors; Janus is to a certain extent their deity, looking back to a ramification of roots and associations and forward to a clarification of sense and meaning.[10]

And he describes the poet as being credited:

with a power to open unexpected and unedited communications between our nature and the nature of the reality we inhabit.[11]

Robert Frost asserts that the true poem:

> ends in a clarification of life – not necessarily a great clarification, such as sects and cults are founded on, but in a momentary stay against confusion.

Sometimes, working together, the doctor and the patient can also find the understanding and the words to provide this momentary stay against confusion and, in so doing, much relief of suffering.

Novelists, too, have much to offer doctors. Our experience of humanity is expanded with each patient contact, but in reading a novel we are offered aspects of the same human experience given breadth and depth by the expressive ability of the writer, which are the same dimensions which we seek to pursue with our patients. Reading, we come across passages which invoke particular individual patients and allow us to see and understand them at a new depth. For example, in *The Conservationist*, Nadine Gordimer writes:

> Distress is a compulsion to examine minutely – this anguished restless necessity, when something can't be undone, when there's nothing to be done, to keep going over and over the same ground.

This is a perfectly precise description of the futile repetitiveness of regret and it has given me a form of words which I have been able to use to show the patient who is trapped in this distress that their suffering is understood.

Those of us lucky enough to lead lives of personal good fortune need writers to make us understand the reality of lives of privation and loss. Novelists can also help us across boundaries, take us into other cultures and provide us with insight into the experience of patients struggling to survive and communicate across barriers of language and culture.

> Lily herself enjoyed good health; fortunately for both of them, she often thought. Until Man Kee had arrived neither had been to a doctor in their time in the UK. Some of the other restaurant employees went to a Cantonese-speaking Indian doctor in Southall if they were seriously ill. But Lily, even now, still felt it mildly disgraceful to take something for nothing.

Chen was also puzzled by this business of registering and form-filling. He had once seen a medical card. The size of the number had been enough to intimidate him.

Timothy Mo
Sour Sweet

Novels tell us stories and those stories resonate to a greater or lesser extent with our own, but the most potent and disturbing resonances are to be found in myth. George Steiner[12] raises the possibility that the power and persistence of the primordial myths derive from their origin alongside the development of language, of the way we use words. He argues:

That mythology and the bone-structure of syntax are somehow interwoven.

As an example he speculates that the invention of future tenses:

might correspond to the invention of hope, of certain tools and techniques of anticipatory cultivation – the sowing of seed towards a subsequent harvest.

He continues:

Nothing is more astounding in our resources of syntax than the evolution of optatives, of subjunctives, of counter-factual propositions. What complex worlds of reasoned imagining underwrite sentences beginning with 'if': if Napoleon had won at Waterloo, if we discover a remedy to Aids, if there had been no Mozart. Such sentences say 'No' to reality, they allow us to inhabit manifold orders of possibility, to dream argumentatively.

In this way, myths give us our most powerful metaphors, a guide to the exploration of our deepest, most ancient and most disturbing feelings, and clues in the search for meaning in human illness.

This century has seen the first literate generations to grow up within Western culture without an intimate knowledge of these myths. At school, I resented deeply being obliged to learn Latin and was relieved not to be force-fed Classical Greek, but I now regret my lack of familiarity with the stories. Why did we stop telling the stories when we stopped learning the archaic languages? We have lost the mythological framework which has the potential to give universality to our individual experience and we are the poorer for it.[13] Mary Midgeley writes:

> We understand today that it is a bad idea to exterminate the natural fauna of the human gut. But trying to exterminate the natural fauna and flora of the human imagination is perhaps no more sensible. We have a choice of what myths, what visions we will use to help us understand the physical world. We do not have a choice of understanding it without using any myths or visions at all. Again, we have a real choice between becoming aware of these myths and ignoring them. If we ignore them, we travel blindly inside myths and visions which are largely provided by other people. This makes it much harder to know where we are going.

The ancient myths range across the whole of human aspiration, from the most noble to the most base, but always valuing the intensity of life more than its length.[14] They tell us all we need to know to make sense of the risks our patients take and the price they are prepared to pay for those risks. Set in this dense context, the emptiness of much health promotion rhetoric is plain.

PARTISANSHIP, PHILOSOPHY AND POLITICS

The general practitioner must strive to be always, vehemently, on the side of the individual patient, witnessing, and sometimes interpreting, their distress. Only by seeking to identify fully with the patient's predicament can the doctor understand. Through this process of empathic identification, the doctor is engaged to serve as the patient's advocate. Edmund Pellegrino[15] has argued the philosophical basis of this position:

> It is not just that Hippocratic professional ethics lacks a theory of just distribution; it is rather that it is committed to the proposition that societal goods do not count ethically. The commitment of the clinician is not just primarily to the patient, it is fully patient-centered. Considering the common good is not an add-on; it is morally wrong.

The role of individual advocate underpins all else, but the general practitioner combines this with a wider social and political responsibility to speak out on behalf of the most needy and least heard. Robin Downle, seeking to answer the evaluative question of what enables professions to perform a unique and socially valuable function, distinct from business and commerce, describes six characteristics of a profession.[16] The third of these involves the duty to speak out on matters of social justice and social utility. Illustrating this characteristic, he writes:

> Doctors have a duty to speak out on broad issues of health, as for example they might speak out against cigarette advertising or cast doubt on the feasibility of medical services in the event of a nuclear attack.

General practitioners are in a privileged position to develop an intimate knowledge of their patients' lives. Those working in areas of socio-economic deprivation are made acutely and repeatedly aware of how squalid overcrowded housing conditions, homelessness, unemployment and poverty undermine the autonomy, dignity, self-respect and health of those who suffer them[17] We see, every day, how society functions in a way which systematically undermines the health of its most vulnerable members. We have a duty to speak out about this because it represents a denial of social justice.[18] Further, we have a responsibility to contribute to the research which makes the links between health and socio-economic conditions explicit and to disseminate that research throughout society. If we can define the social conditions which cause ill health, we begin to define the social changes which will prevent and treat it.[19] We should not shirk that responsibility. I have argued that the general practitioner has the responsibility to approach each individual patient with unconditional positive regard and to become his or her advocate in the face of illness. Equally, the general practitioner has a responsibility to serve as an advocate for those whose health is chronically undermined, either by disease or by their adverse life circumstances. Only in this way can equity be achieved and Julian Tudor Hart's Inverse Care Law[20] be reversed.

TIME, TRUST AND 'THE MATERIALISTIC MIRE OF MARKET MEDICINE'[21]

As general practitioners, we can do nothing for our patients if we lack time to spend with them and if we fail to gain and retain their trust. Time and trust are fundamental to our endeavours and both are being undermined in the current crisis. The demands of health promotion, patient care which was previously undertaken in hospital, care in the community and purchasing in the NHS market, all seriously undermine the availability of time to be spent with patients. The conflict, between the doctor's role as an advocate for the individual patient and his or her increasing responsibility for the allocation of scarce resources across a population, threatens to undermine the trust of patients. With the introduction of market values into the National Health Service, doctors have colluded in arguments that resources for health are necessarily insufficient and have been seduced into accepting responsibility for decisions about the allocation of these scarce resources. However, such decisions are not medical but political and they should be taken by those members of society who can be held democratically accountable for them. The individual patient seeking the advice of a general practitioner must be able to believe that the doctor is acting entirely in that patient's interest. As soon as the patient begins to suspect that a test or a hospital referral is being withheld for budgetary reasons and not because it is unnecessary the patient's trust will be lost and the whole cost-effectiveness of British general practice will evaporate. Patients will insist on inappropriate interventions because they are afraid and the general practitioner, having lost the patient's trust, will be unable to reassure them. Once lost trust will be immensely difficult to regain.

I have described two key but apparently undervalued roles of general practice and I have attempted to show that there are certain requirements for the effective performance of these roles. In discussing these requirements I have been brought back to some of the components of the current crisis because these are threatening the essential prerequisites of good practice.

NOTES AND REFERENCES

1 Midgeley M. *Science as Salvation: a modern myth and its meaning.* London: Routledge, 1992.

'And since people's deepest ideas about the meaning or meaninglessness of life are largely forged in everyday life and in the arts, we would surely do well to pay serious attention to these wherever we can find them.'

2 Sanders K. *Nine Lives: the emotional experience in general practice.* The Roland Harris Education Trust, 1991.

'. . . the courage and the imagination to permit a marriage between art and science. When they are separated, both remain sterile. In combination, they complement one another in an enhanced desire to find meaning in the experience of being alive.'

3 Holmes R. *Footsteps: adventures of a romantic biographer.* London: Hodder and Stoughton, 1985.

4 Kleinman A. *The Illness Narratives: suffering, healing and the human condition.* New York: Basic Books, 1988.

'Another core clinical task is the empathetic interpretation of a life story that makes over the illness into the subject matter of a biography. Here the clinician listens to the sick individual's personal myth, a story that gives shape to an illness so as to distance an otherwise fearsome reality. The clinician attends to the patient's and family's summation of life's trials. Their narrative highlights core life themes – for example, injustice, courage, personal victory against the odds –for whose prosecution the details of illness supply evidence.'

5 Wynne-Jones M. General practice: a job for life? *British Medical Journal.* 1993; 307: 630.

'I left patients with whom I shared an irreplaceable past, underestimating its importance. Changing practices means throwing away the investment of many years' effort.'

6 Berger J and Mohr J. *A Fortunate Man: the story of a country doctor.* Harmondsworth: Allen Lane, The Penguin Press, 1967.

'He does more than treat them when they are ill; he is the objective witness of their lives . . . He keeps the records so that, from time to time, they can consult them themselves . . . He represents them, becomes their objective (as opposed to subjective) memory, because he represents their lost possibility of understanding and relating to the outside world, and because he also represents some of what they know but cannot think.'

7 Marinker M. *The end of general practice*. Bayliss Lecture. London: Royal College of Physicians, 1994.

8 Ignatieff M. *The Needs of Strangers*. London: Chatto & Windus, 1984.

9 Heaney S. *The Government of the Tongue*. London: Faber and Faber, 1988.

10 Heaney S. *Preoccupations: Selected Prose 1968–1978*. London: Faber and Faber, 1980.

11 Quoted in: Heaney S. *The Government of the Tongue*. London: Faber and Faber, 1988.

12 Steiner G. *The Europe Myth*. Salzburger: Festspiele, 1994.

13 Berger J and Mohr J. *A Fortunate Man: the story of a country doctor*. Harmondsworth: Allen Lane, The Penguin Press, 1967.
   'The culturally deprived have far fewer ways of recognising themselves. A great deal of their experience – especially emotional and introspective experience – has to remain unnamed for them.'

14 Calasso R. *The Marriage of Cadmus and Harmony*. London: Jonathan Cape, 1993.
   'The Greeks had no inclination for temperance. They knew that excess is divine, and that the divine overwhelms life. But the more they found themselves immersed in the divine, the more they wished to keep it at arm's length. Western sobriety, which two thousand years later would become everyman's common sense, was at first no more than a mirage glimpsed through the tempest of the elements.'

15 Veatch RM. Justice in health care: the contribution of Edmund Pellegrino. *J Med Phil*. 1990; **15**: 269–87.

16 Downie RS. Professions and professionalism. *J Phil Educ*. 1990; **24**: 147–59.

17 Bartley M. Health costs of social injustice. *British Medical Journal*. 1994; **309**: 1177–8.

18 Watt GCM. Health implications of putting value added tax on fuel. *British Medical Journal*. 1994; **309**: 1030–1.

19 Kleinman A. *The Illness Narratives: suffering, healing and the human condition*. New York: Basic Books, 1988.
   'Both cancer and heart disease intensify our awareness of the dangers of our times and of the man-made sources of much misery. But the governmental response is

meant to obfuscate this vision of sickness as meaning something is wrong with the social order and to replace (medicalize) it with narrowly technical questions. Is there a better mirror of what we are about?'

20 Hart JT. The Inverse Care Law. *Lancet.* 1971; i: 405–12.

21 Morell D. *Diagnosis in General Practice: art or science?* London: Nuffield Provincial Hospitals Trust, 1993.

6 THE FUTURE

I have argued that the general practitioner has two key roles: one as an interpreter and guardian at the interface between illness and disease, the other as witness to the human experience of, and search for meaning in, both illness and disease. The first is a role which belongs to general practice, the second is shared with our specialist colleagues, although continuity of care over time gives much more scope for it in general practice. I have attempted to show that these two roles justify the continuation of general practice in its present form, and that we should not allow them to be displaced, and the nature of general practice changed fundamentally, by the multiplicity of new roles we are being invited to try. Carl Edvard Rudebeck[1] asserts, rightly:

> Beliefs do not convince opponents, especially if these see a danger of losing resources. Logical arguments, catching the specific contribution of general practice to medicine and uniting the individual practitioners into a distinct profession, are essential.

The first key role is easier to justify by logical argument. Although less well understood than the role of gatekeeper to expensive secondary care, it is the other major component of the cost-effectiveness of British general practice. By identifying illness, a sense of bodily unease, as being due to distress rather than disease, we spare the individual patient unnecessary anxiety, tests and treatment, and also save the health service the financial costs of these.

The second role is harder to justify because, as John Berger has argued,[2] its value depends, at least in part, on the worth we attach to an ordinary human life:

> we in our society do not know how to acknowledge, to measure the contribution of an ordinary working doctor . . . when we imaginatively try to take the measure of a man doing no more and no less than easing – and occasionally saving – the lives of a few thousand of our contemporaries. Naturally we count it in principle, a good thing. But fully to take the measure of it, we have to come to some conclusion about the value of these lives to us now . . . I do not claim to know what human life is worth – the question cannot be answered by word but only by action, by the creation of

a more humane society. All that I do know is that our present society wastes and, by the slow draining process of enforced hypocrisy, empties most of the lives which it does not destroy: and that, within its own terms, a doctor who has passed the stage of selling cures, either directly to the patient or through the agency of a state service, is unassessable.

All this is true and is part of the difficulty that we have in justifying ourselves and that our society has in valuing what we have to offer. There is an urgent need to debate these matters, to come to a view as to how highly we should all value the complex tasks of making the human experience of illness and disease less lonely. But first we have to rediscover a set of values which go beyond the numerical and the financial.

Meanwhile, there are other potential benefits in the careful witnessing of the processes of illness and disease. Our patients' stories contain the secrets, the mysteries, of the beginning of illness and within that the beginning of disease. The great contribution of general practice in the future may be in qualitative research,[3] developing what David Metcalfe describes as the 'rigorous qualitative methods [which] are needed to elucidate the 'why' of situations described in quantitative terms'. Much general practice research has suffered through seeking the approbation of specialist colleagues in academic medicine. The task ahead will demand more breadth and flexibility in the definition of academic respectability which is still embedded in the requirements of scientific biomechanical medicine. As Rudebeck states:

> According to this view, an answer should be numeric, otherwise it is not a real answer. If, on the other hand, research is looked upon as an activity adding to or changing our prevailing comprehension of reality through the refinement of observations or experience, then the range of issues may be considerably widened . . . The evaluation of the quality of research at one instant and according to very strict formal criteria which may seem necessary from editorial points of view, is somewhat contradictory to the process of knowledge production itself.

I have argued that the complex mysterious depths of general practice fulfil functions which are beneficial both to individual patients and to the wider cause of human endeavour. Some contend that the wider dissemination of medical knowledge through the application of information technology, combined with the rise of consumerism within a less hierarchical, although perversely more socio-economically divided, society, will change fundamentally the relationship between doctor and patient.[4] However, the demands and rights which drive the consumer relationship offer little prospect of containing the expressed or hidden fears which are implicit in almost every medical encounter.[5] Likewise any doctor who has faced serious illness knows that medical knowledge is similarly ineffective.

On the other hand, it seems certain that the rapid progress of medical technology will mean that it will be possible to deliver closer to patients' homes complex treatments which were previously available only in hospitals. This could be done by enabling specialists to work outside hospitals while retaining a clear-cut referral process. The danger is that it will be done by taking work away from specialists and overloading general practitioners. If this happens, general practitioners will no longer have the time to serve as guardians of the interface between illness and disease or indeed, as gatekeepers between primary and secondary care, with the result that the whole basis of the cost-effectiveness of the UK system of health care will disappear.

The effects of the current changes are enormously destructive. Yet people are beginning to talk of 'change fatigue' and to argue that even if things are bad, nothing radical should be done to remedy the situation because further change could not be endured. This cannot be right. Many of us believe deeply that the recent changes have been at best misguided, and at worst malevolent. We are holding out for a better, more compassionate, future. If the present situation is destructive and will continue to be so, we must seek to work with policy-makers and patients to rectify it.

General practice is a power for good but it is threatened by the process of accelerating change and will only have a future if it can explain and justify itself. There is an urgent need for the value of the key roles to be discussed with students,[6] young doctors and the society we all seek to serve. Only through teaching do we make our own understanding explicit.[7] Without sharing that understanding, we risk losing something immensely precious.

NOTES AND REFERENCES

1 Rudebeck CE. General practice and the dialogue of clinical practice: on symptoms, symptom presentations and bodily empathy. *Scand J Prim Health Care.* 1992; **Suppl 1.**

2 Berger J and Mohr J. *A Fortunate Man: the story of a country doctor.* Harmondsworth: Allen Lane, The Penguin Press, 1967.

3 Murphy E and Mattson B. Qualitative research and family practice: a marriage made in heaven? *Fam Pract.* 1992; 9: 85–91.

4 Kernick DP. General practice's last stand. *British Medical Journal.* 1995; 310: 1613.

5 Thomasma DC. Establishing the moral basis of medicine: Edmund D Pellegrino's philosophy of medicine. *J Med Phil.* 1990; 15: 245–67.
'. . . the instinctive resistance practising physicians often have towards over-emphasizing autonomy in the doctor–patient relationship. One cannot abandon persons to their autonomy when they are in difficult straits.'

6 Marinker M. 2010. *J R Coll Gen Pract.* 1981; 31: 540–6.

7 Stevens J. Brief encounter. *J Roy Coll Gen Pract.* 1974; 24: 5–22.